Current Perspectives on Management of Calcaneal Fractures

Editor

THOMAS S. ROUKIS

CLINICS IN PODIATRIC MEDICINE AND SURGERY

www.podiatric.theclinics.com

Consulting Editor
THOMAS J. CHANG

April 2019 • Volume 36 • Number 2

ELSEVIER

1600 John F. Kennedy Boulevard • Suite 1800 • Philadelphia, Pennsylvania, 19103-2899

http://www.theclinics.com

CLINICS IN PODIATRIC MEDICINE AND SURGERY Volume 36, Number 2
April 2019 ISSN 0891-8422, ISBN-13: 978-0-323-67821-6

Editor: Lauren Boyle
Developmental Editor: Sara Watkins

Clinics in Podiatric Medicine and Surgery (ISSN 0891-8422) is published quarterly by Elsevier Inc., 360 Park Avenue South, New York, NY 10010-1710. Months of issue are January, April, July, and October. Business and Editorial Offices: 1600 John F. Kennedy Blvd., Ste. 1800, Philadelphia, PA 19103-2899. Customer Service Office: 3251 Riverport Lane, Maryland Heights, MO 63043. Periodicals postage paid at New York, NY and additional mailing offices. Subscription prices are $304.00 per year for US individuals, $574.00 per year for US institutions, $100.00 per year for US students and residents, $382.00 per year for Canadian individuals, $693.00 for Canadian institutions, $439.00 for international individuals, $693.00 per year for international institutions and $220.00 per year for Canadian and foreign students/residents. To receive student/resident rate, orders must be accompanied by name of affiliated institution, date of term, and the *signature* of program/residency coordinator on institution letterhead. Orders will be billed at individual rate until proof of status is received. Foreign air speed delivery is included in all *Clinics* subscription prices. All prices are subject to change without notice. POSTMASTER: Send address changes to *Clinics in Podiatric Medicine and Surgery*, Elsevier Health Sciences Division, Subscription Customer Service, 3251 Riverport Lane, Maryland Heights, MO 63043. **Customer Service: 1-800-654-2452 (US). From outside of the US, call 314-447-8871. Fax: 314-447-8029. E-mail: JournalsCustomerService-usa@elsevier.com (for print support); JournalsOnlineSupport-usa@elsevier. com (for online support).**

Reprints. For copies of 100 or more of articles in this publication, please contact the Commercial Reprints Department, Elsevier Inc., 360 Park Avenue South, New York, NY 10010-1710. Tel.: 212-633-3874; Fax: 212-633-3820; E-mail: reprints@elsevier.com.

Clinics in Podiatric Medicine and Surgery is covered in *MEDLINE/PubMed (Index Medicus)* and *EMBASE/Excerpta Medica*.

Contributors

CONSULTING EDITOR

THOMAS J. CHANG, DPM
Clinical Professor and Past Chairman, Department of Podiatric Surgery, California College of Podiatric Medicine, Faculty, The Podiatry Institute, Redwood Orthopedic Surgery Associates, Santa Rosa, California, USA

EDITOR

THOMAS S. ROUKIS, DPM, PhD, FACFAS
Attending Staff, Orthopaedic Center, Gundersen Health System, La Crosse, Wisconsin, USA

AUTHORS

CHRISTOPHER BIBBO, DO, DPM, FACS, FACFAS, FAAOS
Chief, Foot and Ankle Section, Plastic Reconstructive and Microsurgery, Musculoskeletal Infection Service, Limb Salvage, and Orthopaedic Trauma, Rubin Institute for Advanced Orthopaedics, Sinai Hospital of Baltimore, Baltimore, Maryland, USA

GABRIEL CELLARIER, MD
Institut Pied & Cheville, Centre Hospitalier d'Agen, Agen, France

JAMES M. COTTOM, DPM
Director, Florida Orthopedic Foot and Ankle Center Fellowship, Sarasota, Florida, USA

MARISSA S. DAVID, DPM
Podiatric Surgery Resident (PGY-III), Kaiser Permanente Santa Clara and GSAA, Santa Clara, California, USA

STEVEN M. DOUTHETT, DPM
Oregon Medical Group, Eugene, Oregon, USA

DAVID A. EHRLICH, MD
Reconstructive and Plastic Surgery, Private Practice, Philadelphia, Pennsylvania, USA

JESSICA FINK, DPM
Foot and Ankle Deformity and Orthoplastics Fellow, Rubin Institute for Advanced Orthopaedics, Sinai Hospital of Baltimore, Baltimore, Maryland, USA

DIDIER FUENTES-VIEJO, MD, PhD
Institut Pied & Cheville, Centre Hospitalier d'Agen, Agen, France

BRENT A. FUERBRINGER, DPM
Attending Staff, Podiatric Medicine and Surgery Department, Gundersen Healthcare System, Tomah, Wisconsin, USA

PETER J. HORDYK, DPM
Attending Staff, Podiatric Medicine and Surgery Department, Gundersen Healthcare System, Tomah, Wisconsin, USA

KELLI L. ICEMAN, DPM
PGY-3, Podiatric Medicine and Surgery Resident, Gundersen Medical Foundation, La Crosse, Wisconsin, USA

STEVEN J. KOVACH, MD
Assistant Professor, Plastic Reconstructive and Orthopaedic Surgery, University of Pennsylvania Health System, Perelman Center for Advanced Medicine, Philadelphia, Pennsylvania, USA

TRAPPER LALLI, MD
Assistant Professor, Department of Orthopaedic Surgery, The University of Texas Southwestern Medical Center, Dallas, Texas, USA

ADAM LANDSMAN, DPM, PhD
Chief, Division of Podiatric Surgery, Cambridge Health Alliance, Assistant Professor of Surgery, Harvard Medical School, Cambridge, Massachusetts, USA

PHILIEN LAUER
Department of Trauma, Hand and Reconstructive Surgery, Rostock University Medical Center, Rostock, Germany

GEORGE T. LIU, DPM, FACFAS
Associate Professor, Department of Orthopaedic Surgery, The University of Texas Southwestern Medical Center, Dallas, Texas, USA

TUN-HING LUI, MBBS (HK), FRCS (Edin), FHKAM, FHKCOS
Department of Orthopaedics and Traumatology, North District Hospital, Hong Kong SAR, China

MARK K. MAGNUS, DPM
PGY-3, Podiatric Medicine and Surgery Resident, Gundersen Medical Foundation, La Crosse, Wisconsin, USA

KELLY K. McCONNELL, DPM
Coastline Foot and Ankle Center, Salem, Oregon, USA

GARRETT MELICK, DPM
Second Year Podiatric Surgical Resident, Cambridge Health Alliance, Cambridge, Massachusetts, USA

THOMAS MITTLMEIER, MD, PhD
Chair, Department of Trauma, Hand and Reconstructive Surgery, Rostock University Medical Center, Rostock, Germany

XIAO-HUA PAN, MD
Guangdong Provincial Engineering Research Center of Wound Repair and Regenerative Medicine, Guangdong Provincial Academician Workstation of Wound Repair and Regenerative Medicine, Department of Trauma and Orthopedics, Affiliated Baoan Hospital of Shenzhen, Southern Medical University, The 8th People's Hospital of Shenzhen, Shenzhen, Guangdong, China

YU PAN, MD
Guangdong Provincial Engineering Research Center of Wound Repair and Regenerative Medicine, Guangdong Provincial Academician Workstation of Wound Repair and Regenerative Medicine, Department of Trauma and Orthopedics, Affiliated Baoan Hospital of Shenzhen, Southern Medical University, The 8th People's Hospital of Shenzhen, Shenzhen, Guangdong, China

CHUL HYUN PARK, MD, PhD
Associate Professor, Department of Orthopedic Surgery, Yeungnam University Medical Center, Daegu, Republic of Korea

JAKE POWERS, DPM
Chief Resident, Sinai Hospital of Baltimore, Baltimore, VA, Foot and Ankle Surgery Residency, Baltimore, Maryland, USA

ANUSHA PUNDU, DPM
First Year Podiatric Surgical Resident, Cambridge Health Alliance, Cambridge, Massachusetts, USA

KATHERINE M. RASPOVIC, DPM, FACFAS
Assistant Professor, Department of Orthopaedic Surgery, The University of Texas Southwestern Medical Center, Dallas, Texas, USA

THOMAS S. ROUKIS, DPM, PhD, FACFAS
Attending Staff, Orthopaedic Center, Gundersen Health System, La Crosse, Wisconsin, USA

TIM SCHEPERS, MD, PhD
Trauma Surgeon, Trauma Unit, Amsterdam UMC, Amsterdam Movement Sciences, Amsterdam, The Netherlands

NOMAN SIDDIQUI, DPM, MHA
Division Chief of Podiatric Surgery at Northwest Hospital, Director, Diabetic Limb Preservation at Lifebridge Health, Fellowship Director of Foot and Ankle Service, Rubin Institute for Advanced Orthopaedics, Sinai Hospital of Baltimore, Baltimore, Maryland, USA

PATRICK SIMON, MD, PhD
Clinical Professor, Lyon, France

MITCHELL J. THOMPSON, DPM
PGY-2, Podiatric Medicine and Surgery Resident, Gundersen Medical Foundation, La Crosse, Wisconsin, USA

MICHAEL D. VANPELT, DPM, FACFAS
Associate Professor, Department of Orthopaedic Surgery, The University of Texas Southwestern Medical Center, Dallas, Texas, USA

GLENN M. WEINRAUB, DPM, FACFAS
Co-Director, KP Global Health-Vietnam Project, GME Dir., TPMG-GSAA, Attending Staff, Department of Orthopaedic Surgery, San Leandro, California, USA; Clinical Assistant Professor, Midwestern University, Glendale, Arizona, USA; Clinical Associate Professor, Western University, Pomona, California, USA; Past President, Fellow, American College of Foot and Ankle Surgeons, Chicago, Illinois, USA

DANE K. WUKICH, MD
Professor, Department of Orthopaedic Surgery, The University of Texas Southwestern Medical Center, Dallas, Texas, USA

Contents

should play a significant role in planning the surgical incision, and may dictate the repair options available to the surgeon.

Although open reduction and internal fixation for treating displaced intra-articular calcaneal fractures remain common, difficulty obtaining and maintaining both calcaneal morphology and subtalar articular surface reduction remain. In addition, open approaches induce a significant risk of wound-healing complications. For this reason, closed manipulation to restore calcaneal morphology, intra-osseous fracture reduction, and rigid locked nail fixation was developed and validated for clinical use. Conversion to an immediate primary or delayed reconstructive subtalar joint arthrodesis using the same instrumentation remains unique to this system. This article reviews the CALCANAIL surgical technique for performing operative fixation of displaced intra-articular calcaneal fractures.

Treatment of displaced intra-articular calcaneal fractures has changed numerous times in the last decades. Currently, less invasive surgery has reemerged and is increasingly used. The sinus tarsi approach is most commonly used. It combines the open approach to the subtalar joint with percutaneous reduction of the overall shape of the calcaneus. The results in the literature show overall similar functional outcome compared with the extended lateral approach, however with a significant reduction in wound complications. This article deals with the sinus tarsi approach in which the reduction is fixated using screws only. Indications, surgical technique, and possible pitfalls are discussed.

 Video content accompanies this article at http://www.podiatric. theclinics.com.

Displaced intra-articular calcaneal fractures can be treated with open reduction and internal fixation through various methods, including the extensile lateral approach, sinus tarsi approach, percutaneous reduction and fixation, external fixation, and calcaneoplasty. Although the gold standard is the extensile lateral approach, this method has significant wound-healing complications associated with it. Literature shows that the reduction achieved through minimally invasive techniques is equal to that achieved with the extensile lateral approach, while reducing the amount of postoperative complications. This article outlines a technique that uses the sinus tarsi approach with subcutaneous plate fixation.

Subtalar arthroscopy has an important role in enhancing the reduction of the posterior facet in percutaneous and open approaches of displaced intra-articular calcaneal fractures. In the percutaneous approach, arthroscopically assistant percutaneous approach must be selected carefully for mild-to-moderately displaced fractures. In the open approach, there is still little evidence of the utility of subtalar arthroscopy. Therefore, intraoperative arthroscopy should always be used in conjunction with fluoroscopy to achieve reduction and assess the internal fixation placement.

Displaced intra-articular calcaneal fractures represent life-altering injuries. Difficulty obtaining and maintaining calcaneal morphology and the significant risk of wound healing complications with an extensile lateral incision exist. Open reduction with internal fixation as a joint-sparing approach has been studied. Closed manipulation to restore calcaneal morphology, intraosseous fracture reduction, and rigid locked CALCANAIL fracture nail fixation have recently been applied to Sanders IV fracture patterns. Spontaneous conversion to primary subtalar joint arthrodesis using the same instrumentation remains unique to this system. This article reviews open and percutaneous approaches for joint-sparing and primary arthrodesis procedures to treat Sanders IV fracture patterns.

Fractures of the calcaneus are detrimental injuries, often caused by high-energy trauma. To best restore the functionality of a limb and allow normal ambulation, it is recommended to repair displaced intra-articular calcaneus fractures surgically. This article presents several methods of reduction and repair of the calcaneus. Traditionally, calcaneal fractures have been repaired through a lateral extensile incision that has been shown to have a high percentage of wound healing complications. In recent times, there has been a shift toward minimally invasive and sinus tarsi incisional approaches in the repair of calcaneus fractures.

The list of late complications after calcaneal fracture that can be treated through arthroscopic and/or endoscopic approach continues to expand. The late complications of calcaneal fractures can be classified into 3 groups: (1) those causing focal hindfoot or ankle pain, (2) those causing functional deficit, and (3) those present with diffuse and poorly localized pain. Many group 1 and some group 2 complications can be managed arthroscopically and/or endoscopically. There are usually multiple coexisting

Kelli L. Iceman, Mark K. Magnus, and Thomas S. Roukis

A subset of calcaneal fractures is so severe that it may warrant primary conservative treatment. Unfortunately, nonoperative management of these fractures can lead to the development of a calcaneal malunion and cause significant patient morbidity. Surgical management of these deformities often requires increasingly complex reconstructive procedures. The goals of surgery include re-establishing calcaneal height, restoring the talocalcaneal relationship, and creating a stable, plantigrade foot. This article highlights the available surgical treatment options (including calcanectomy, calcaneal allograft transplantation, vascularized autografts, and calcaneal prostheses) for the management of severe calcaneal malunion deformities.

CLINICS IN PODIATRIC MEDICINE AND SURGERY

ISSUE OF RELATED INTEREST

Foot and Ankle Clinics, October 2013 (Vol. 23, No. 1)
Management of Metatarsalgia and Painful Lesser Toe Deformities
Todd A. Irwin, *Editor*
Available at: https://www.foot.theclinics.com/

Foreword

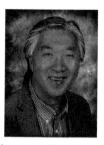

Thomas J. Chang, DPM
Consulting Editor

It is a pleasure to present this next issue, which offers an up-to-date dissection on all aspects of Calcaneal fracture management. There are few lower-extremity conditions we encounter that may dramatically affect one's return to a functional quality of life as these injuries do. When the primary injury, or the neglected fracture, or postinjury complications are considered, both surgical and nonsurgical, these all pose potential life-altering affects on our patients.

Dr Roukis has dedicated part of his career to carefully evaluating and processing the foot and ankle literature on certain topics to share the pertinent conclusions with us. In his meta-analysis of many topic areas, he has found a paucity of recent publications on the topic of calcaneal fractures. Throughout his career, he has gained tremendous experience with this deformity. Coupled with his flair for education and publications, he has been able to contribute significantly to current management concepts of this deformity. I feel this topic is timely, and this may soon be considered the most complete collection of articles put together on Calcaneal fractures for many years to come.

As always, I thank Dr Roukis and his list of respected authors for their time and the efforts put into this project. I hope you will find it meaningful. I know I will.

Thomas J. Chang, DPM
Redwood Orthopedic Surgery Associates
208 Concourse Boulevard
Santa Rosa, CA 95403, USA

E-mail address:
thomaschang14@comcast.net

Clin Podiatr Med Surg 36 (2019) xiii
https://doi.org/10.1016/j.cpm.2018.11.002
0891-8422/19/© 2018 Published by Elsevier Inc.

Preface

Contemporary Management of Displaced Intra-Articular Calcaneal Fractures

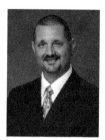

Thomas S. Roukis, DPM, PhD, FACFAS
Editor

It is with great pleasure that I serve as Guest Editor for this issue of *Clinics in Podiatric Medicine and Surgery* devoted to "Current Perspectives on Management of Calcaneal Fractures." Surprisingly few textbooks or *Clinics in Podiatric Medicine and Surgery* issues devoted entirely to calcaneal fractures exist, and many of those that do are outdated or involve fixation systems that are not available for use in the United States. The authors selected for this issue are respected authorities on the topics they have been assigned, and they have been gracious enough to take substantial time from their practices and families to accommodate my tight, and in many ways unrealistic, goals for this issue.

The intent of the issue is to help solve some of the mysteries associated with this "unsolved" intra-articular injury and refute the idea that it is "unsolvable." To do so, we start with a detailed review of the initial management considerations for acute injuries and then turn our attention to a number of controversies, surgical approaches, and fixation options germane to our current understanding of calcaneal fractures. A detailed review of specialized techniques useful for addressing the frustrating common complications that develop postoperatively, including nonunion, malunion, and wounding, follows. We conclude with our current options and future perspective on salvaging the unsalvageable calcaneal malunion deformity.

Clin Podiatr Med Surg 36 (2019) xv–xvi
https://doi.org/10.1016/j.cpm.2018.11.001
0891-8422/19/© 2018 Published by Elsevier Inc.

podiatric.theclinics.com

It is hoped that the readers of this issue of *Clinics of Podiatric Medicine and Surgery* will enjoy these articles and benefit from the surgical experience of the authors selected as much as I have.

Thomas S. Roukis, DPM, PhD, FACFAS
Gundersen Health System
Orthopaedic Center
Mail Stop: CO2-006
1900 South Avenue
La Crosse, WI 54601-5467, USA

E-mail address:
tsroukis@gundersenhealth.org

Clinical Management of Acute, Closed Displaced Intra-Articular Calcaneal Fractures

Peter J. Hordyk, DPM[a], Brent A. Fuerbringer, DPM[a], Thomas S. Roukis, DPM, PhD[b],*

KEYWORDS

- Calcaneus • Clinical examination • Clinical management
- Concurrent considerations • Trauma

KEY POINTS

- Clinical assessment necessitates management of the osseous and soft tissue injury.
- Initial therapy should focus on edema reduction, pain control, and preoperative optimization.
- Protocol-driven practices with clear guidelines can prevent morbidity and increase compliance.
- Appropriate clinical management prevents delayed operative intervention and improves outcomes.

INTRODUCTION

Displaced intra-articular calcaneal fractures (DIACF) are substantial injuries associated with prolonged incapacitation. Initial management is complex and its importance to the ultimate outcome is often understated. Proper initial identification, evaluation, and treatment are imperative to ensure the ideal outcome. To provide optimal clinical management, there must be a clear understanding of the pathology, possible sequelae, and confounding social factors. Failure to perform careful assessment and thoughtful initial treatment can increase the risk of morbidity.

These complex fractures result from axillary loading forces with abrupt deceleration.[1,2] The immense forces applied to the bone result in an explosion type injury of the heel with multiple varying fracture patterns. Greater applied force results in increased derangement of osseous structures and increased compromise to

Disclosure Statement: The authors have no relevant financial disclosures.
[a] Podiatric Medicine and Surgery Department, Gundersen Healthcare System, 1330 North Superior Avenue, Tomah, WI 54660, USA; [b] Orthopaedic Center, Gundersen Health System, Mail Stop: CO2-006, 1900 South Avenue, La Crosse, WI 54601, USA
* Corresponding author.
E-mail address: tsroukis@gundersenhealth.org

Clin Podiatr Med Surg 36 (2019) 163–171
https://doi.org/10.1016/j.cpm.2018.10.001
0891-8422/19/© 2018 Elsevier Inc. All rights reserved.

surrounding soft tissue envelope.[3,4] The unique soft tissue anatomy leads to increased risk of sequelae, such as fracture blisters, soft tissue wounding, and compartment syndrome. Clinical management of acute, closed DIACF should involve management of the osseous fracture and the significant and challenging soft tissue injury.

INITIAL SURVEY

On presentation to the emergency department or urgent care settings, these patients require a complete history and physical work-up given their correlation with high velocity trauma and concomitant injuries, which may take precedence. Initial evaluation of the foot and ankle is focused to rule out any urgent need for intervention. Open fractures and/or compartment syndrome necessitate emergent care. Once emergent needs are ruled out, focus is directed toward the soft tissue, osseous, and often overlooked patient-related social components frequently associated with DIACF.

Individuals with high-energy injuries should be assessed by an emergency medicine or trauma provider to rule out injury to internal organs and proximal osseous structures. Providers should complete a thorough neurologic examination to rule out head and spinal injury. Clinical assessment of the lumbar spine should be performed and careful consideration for radiographic assessment should be weighed. Walters and colleagues[5] in a retrospective cohort study determined that more than 7% of calcaneal fractures are associated with vertebral fracture. After medical clearance and triage is complete initial evaluation of the foot and ankle is commenced.

Close initial survey of the integument should be completed to determine clinical status of the soft tissue envelope. Because of the close association of the underlying osseous structures with the integument it is imperative to assess for open fractures and at-risk integument. Shortening and widening of the calcaneus seen with joint depression–type fractures place pressure to the lateral soft tissues, which can lead to difficult to manage lateral wounding and delay surgical intervention. Similarly, tongue-type fractures can have posterior displacement of the fracture fragment leading to pressure wounding to the posterior heel.[6] Undue pressure to the overlying soft tissue necessitates urgent decompression to avoid further injury. Open fractures to the heel tend to be rare (3%–6%), but should not be overlooked.[7] Open fractures should be managed via a systematic approach with immunization, antibiotic prophylaxis, and irrigation/débridement.[8]

Compartment syndrome develops when the pressure within the small closed soft tissue space increases to the point where blood flow, musculoskeletal, and sensory function is impaired.[4] Incidence is estimated to range from 1% to 10% with calcaneal fractures and have severe sequelae if not properly identified and treated.[9,10] Long-term sequelae include permanent pain, deformity/contracture, weakness, and loss of function. Those who go undiagnosed have been shown to have significantly lower functional outcome scores and are most commonly associated with Sanders type III or IV fracture patterns. Prompt fasciotomy, preferably within 6 hours of onset, has been shown to negate the potential life-altering sequelae.[10] Standard needle manometer system is used to measure and compare pressures within each compartment with 30 mm Hg being the traditional cutoff for operative intervention. Decompression should be pursued despite low readings if there is clinical suspicion secondary to the severe morbidity of undiagnosed compartment syndrome. Findings that should trigger suspicion include tense pedal compartments, persistent paresthesia, and uncontrollable pain.

SECONDARY SURVEY

Following stabilization and medical clearance, a thorough history and systematic examination should be undertaken. A complete history including mechanism and events surrounding the injury should be established. Medical history and medications should be reviewed with the patient to identify any potential barriers to healing. Importantly, the social situation of the patient should be established to assist with treatment planning. A person's social background can pose significant implications on the ultimate treatment course and likelihood of a successful outcome. Social factors that serve as barriers are often underaddressed. These factors play a significant role in the patient's ability to adhere to postoperative protocols and can ultimately lead the patient to further harm. Information regarding the patient's baseline mobility, occupation, transportation, living situation, substance use, and support network should be understood before determining treatment course. Examination should include a thorough clinical appraisal of bilateral lower extremities and radiologic investigation. A protocol-based approach is recommended to prevent omission of vital examination components.

Neurovascular status is established via standard examination. Innervation of lower extremity dermatomes is confirmed with a combination of light touch, sharp/dull provocative testing, and active toe motion. Sensation may be blunted secondary to edema but should remain in place and easy to assess bedside. Vascular status should be established with palpation and hand-held Doppler arterial examination. Medially, the course of the posterior tibial artery should be Dopplerable around the medial malleolus and along the calcaneus into its bifurcating branches and the medial and lateral plantar arteries. Peroneal arterial flow should be examined as described by Bibbo and colleagues[11] tracing the artery proximal and distal to the ankle joint. The examination should be completed with confirmation of patent anterior tibial, dorsalis pedis, and perforating peroneal arteries. Antegrade flow should be confirmed in all tested arteries with a modified Allen test. This is performed by compressing the vessel proximal to the Doppler probe and noting any loss of signal. Failure to detect a Doppler signal is concerning for retrograde flow and subsequent compromised vascular supply.[12] In cases of unilateral injury, findings should be compared with the contralateral extremity because variations in foot and ankle vascular anatomy are common. It is important to understand the baseline vascular status and angiosome distribution for surgical planning.

Musculoskeletal assessment often reveals a shortened and widened calcaneus with visible limb length discrepancy as a result of axillary loading forces.[1,2] Clinical evaluation should involve assessment of the osseous fracture and soft tissue injury. Immense forces are applied to the bone at time of injury that result in osseous derangement. The thin soft tissue envelope is at risk for wounding and thus the heel should be meticulously evaluated for any osseous prominence. Common areas of concern include the lateral heel secondary to lateral wall blowout, medial tarsal canal region because of displacement of the sustentaculum tali and hematoma, and the posterior heel because of displacement of the calcaneal tuber.

Additional musculoskeletal assessment should evaluate for associated injuries. A complete examination of lower extremity osseous structures should be completed to help identify any concomitant injuries. Soft tissue compartments of the foot and ankle should be evaluated to ensure they are soft and supple. Tense compartments should prompt testing with a needle manometer and possible intervention. Evaluation for often overlooked sequelae of calcaneal fractures should be completed including peroneal impingement and or dislocation, which has been associated with calcaneal fractures that involve lateral wall blow-out. It is important to have a high index of suspicion for peroneal involvement.[2,4,13]

Special attention should be paid to the integument. The extent of osseous injury should not overshadow the soft tissue component because it ultimately determines operative timing and outcome. One often notes early onset edema with loss of normal skin lines. Ecchymosis is commonly noted along the plantar arch in a pattern that is pathognomonic of a DIACF. The pattern of ecchymosis to the plantar surface is known as a Mondor sign.

Inspection should be conducted to assess for any abrasions or frank breaches of the integument. During the inspection any at-risk segments should be identified. Formal skin tenting is uncommon; however, because of osseous displacement, diffuse tension to overlying skin is not uncommon. Full-thickness wounding has been shown to occur from inside-out related pressure. Overt concern for impending wounding requires management to allow the soft tissue envelope to recover before definitive fixation.[2]

During initial injury, the integument sustains shear forces that result in damage and subsequently in blister formation. Prevalence is noted to be higher with comminuted fractures.[1,4,14] Although not always present on initial evaluation, fracture blisters are commonly identified in the days following injury as the post-traumatic edema emerges. It has been our experience that strict protocols including scheduling ice, sustained lower limb elevation, and multilayered toes to knee compression dressings aid in overall reduction and severity. The nature of the blisters contents indicates depth of injury. Serous filled blisters retain the protective epidermal cells and risk of infection post-lysis remains low when compared with hemorrhagic blisters. Presence of blood indicates deeper level of involvement, specifically, loss of all epidermal cells.[1,4,14]

IMAGING

Clinical examination should be supplemented with imaging studies to confirm the diagnosis and better understand the nature of the displaced intra-articular fracture. Initial radiographic series are often obtained by emergency medicine providers and usually include non-weight-bearing anterior-posterior, oblique, and lateral radiographs of the foot; anterior-posterior and mortise views of the ankle; and an axial calcaneal view. On referral, noncontrast computed tomography (CT) scans should be ordered for further delineation of calcaneal injury and assistance with identifying concomitant injuries. CT imaging has become the gold standard for evaluation and has replaced the need for specialty views, such as Broden and Harris views on initial evaluation.[4,15] Assessment with CT imaging is recommended because studies have indicated poor correlation between plain radiographic measurements and outcome.[15] Additionally, CT imaging provides a better understanding of fracture pathology, although studies have indicated inconsistent surgeon interpretation of CT findings.[16] Addition of three-dimensional reconstruction to the CT scan allows for added understanding of the pathology and more in depth information for treatment planning. Roll and colleagues[17] in a prospective multicenter study noted improved fracture evaluation with addition of three-dimensional reconstructions compared with standard CT imaging.

INITIAL CLINICAL MANAGEMENT

A well-planned initial evaluation and management of an acute closed DIACF is crucial to allow for ideal surgical timing and optimal outcome. Thorough and systematic evaluation should be followed by a literature-based, protocol-driven, management tailored to patient-specific factors and the nature of the fracture. As with all traumatic injuries measures should be taken to control factors that may hinder treatment including: motion, pain, edema, and thrombosis. Additionally, attempts should be taken to assist with social burdens including time off work, financial concerns, substance abuse, and living environment (**Box 1**).

It is our standard practice to perform soap and water cleansing of the injured extremity during or immediately following evaluation followed by application of a modified Sir Robert Jones dressing with plaster posterior splinting. This serves to ensure proper hygiene and reduce bacterial burden and reduce risk of infection with minimal added cost or effort.[18-20] We then apply a well-padded modified Sir Robert Jones multilayer compression dressing from toes to knee as a means of protecting and stabilizing the extremity while maintaining a consistent level of compression throughout the lower limb.[21] It is our experience that adding several "dressing sandwiches" consisting of cotton padding folded around several gauze[22] that are then placed on the posterior, medial, and lateral heel has reduced pressure-induced wounding and blister formation while affording sustained compression. A plaster short-leg splint is then placed posteriorly with the ankle joint in mild equinus to prevent undue tension across the Achilles and posterior tuber of the calcaneus. Circumferential casting is avoided to prevent dressing-induced compartment syndrome and wounding. Sugar-tong splinting is also avoided because we have anecdotally noted increased lateral wounding secondary to pressure. It is recommended that the most experienced person available be responsible for dressing application to ensure adequate padding and even compression to the already compromised soft tissue envelope.

Box 1
Clinical management checklist

- Initial evaluation
  - Evaluate for other injuries
    - Exclude lumbar spine fracture
    - Exclude contralateral injury
    - Exclude other ipsilateral injury
  - Evaluate for emergent conditions
    - Exclude open fracture
    - Exclude compartment syndrome
    - Exclude at-risk integument

- Secondary evaluation
  - Review medical history and medications
  - Review social history to identify barriers to care
    - Tobacco, alcohol, recreational drugs
    - Occupation/financial situation
    - Place of residence (ie, homeless shelter or second floor bathroom)
    - Support network (transportation and/or assistance at home)
  - Systematic clinical evaluation

- Imaging
  - Baseline radiographs
    - Three-view ankle and foot and axial calcaneal
  - CT imaging with reconstruction

- Initial treatment
  - Cleanse extremity
  - Protect, immobilize, and compress
  - Therapy referral to ensure safe mobilization
  - Initiate ice and elevation protocols
  - Deep vein thrombosis prophylaxis
  - Multimodal pain control
  - Optimization of social situation

When fracture blisters are present it is our practice to lyse and deroof the lesions followed by application of silver sulfadiazine 1% (Pfizer, Inc, New York, NY) and the nonadherent Xeroform petrolatum dressing (Covidien, USA/Medtronics, Minneapolis, MN).[14] The area of concern is offloaded with a folded cotton aperture pad "dressing sandwiches" previously described.[22] We have found the most concerning areas to have complete healing by the day of surgery with the previously mentioned cares.

We prefer to initially admit for pain control and skilled therapies because patients and family members frequently underestimate difficulties with pain control and safe mobilization in the days following injury. In our experience it is safer for the patient to gain initial pain control in an inpatient setting allowing use of adjunctive modalities, such as a popliteal/saphenous nerve lower extremity block and patient-controlled analgesia. Additionally, there is an ability to safely titrate medications and enforce strict bed rest during the acute phase of injury. Patients are educated on in-bed modalities and instructed on use of incentive spirometer for prevention of iatrogenic disease. Over the past decade in our facility we have used a universal lower extremity elevation protocol entailing specific bed positioning and lower extremity elevation as described by Schweinberger and Roukis,[23] which is easily reproducible in the home environment. Elevation is augmented with ice application to the popliteal fossa for 15 minutes each hour awake for improved edema control.[24] Once pain is adequately controlled, patients work with physical and occupational therapy staff for sit-to-stand, turn-and-transfer, and short distance mobilization without "hopping" on the contralateral extremity. These activities ensure safe mobilization while maintaining non-weight-bearing status to the affected extremity. Ultimate placement in a skilled nursing facility or in-patient rehabilitation environment is not uncommon because of patient's physical inability to return home safely.

Pain management is approached via a multimodal technique using narcotic and nonnarcotic analgesia commonly in combination with gabapentinoids. Multimodal pain control has proven effective in limiting narcotic use and provides overall better pain control when compared with monotherapy.[25] Additionally, we have noted that timely application of the modified Sir Robert Jones dressing and posterior plater splint, adherence to strict elevation, and scheduled ice therapy significantly reduce narcotic use. Our preference is to provide multimodal therapies as follows for baseline pain associated with DIACF taken on a scheduled not as needed basis: acetaminophen (Johnson & Johnson, New Brunswick, NJ), 500-mg tablet with two taken by mouth every 8 hours scheduled; Celecoxib (Pfizer, Inc), 200 mg by mouth every 12 hours scheduled; gabapentin (Pfizer, Inc), 300 mg by mouth three times daily; and tramadol (Janssen Pharmaceuticals, Raritan, NJ), 50 to 100 mg by mouth every 8 hours scheduled for baseline pain. Oxycodone HCL (Purdue Pharma, Stamford, CT), 5 to 10 mg by mouth every 4, 6, or 8 hours is used as needed for severe breakthrough pain. Alternative means of pain mitigation, such as essential oils and distraction therapies, are also offered.

Lower extremity trauma has been linked to higher risk of venous thromboembolism with upward of 12% of isolated DIACF sustaining deep vein thrombosis preoperatively.[26,27] It is our protocol to encourage sustained hydration and initiate mechanical and pharmacologic prophylaxis. Mechanical interventions include use of sequential compression devices, contralateral thigh-high TED hose compression, and hourly mobility pending appropriate pain control. In bed exercises are used as an adjunct to mobility and taught to the patient by physical and occupational therapy specialists. Pharmacologic intervention entails enoxaparin (Sanofi US, Bridgewater, NJ), 40 mg subcutaneously once daily for 14 to 21 days depending on the patient's ability to comply with the mechanical protocol and insurance coverage limitations. Once completed, we initiate aspirin (Bayer Corporation, Whippany, NJ), 325 mg by mouth every 12 hours with food. Those at heightened risk for thromboembolism are postoperatively transitioned to a long-term anticoagulant, specifically coumadin (Bristol-Myers Squibb, New York, NY) with specific dosing being controlled by the patient's primary medical provider during the initial 8-week non-weight-bearing period of immobilization. Choice of anticoagulation is based on the patient's medical history and risk profile via Wells criteria[28] and the American College of Foot and Ankle Surgeons Clinical Consensus Statement on thromboembolism disease.[29,30]

Individuals predictably have worse outcome when they are required to stress themselves to safeguard fiscal benefits, fulfill family requirements, and ensure other obligations are upheld. Manual laborers have been linked to having poorer outcomes in general.[4] Not only does this injury set them up for prolonged impaired mobility, but ultimately may prevent return to their skilled trade and require a change in occupation. Thus, taking time to address and ensure their home environment and support network is appropriate is crucial. If not, it may be in their best interest to be placed in a nursing facility for a short term to prevent further complication of the injury and surgery. Social work and financial counselors are enlisted to help arrange discharge to a safe environment and to help enroll patients in programs to alleviate financial concerns. Guidance is provided on use of short-term disability coverage and family and medical leave. Additional consultation is sought to address other social concerns, such as substance abuse. Tobacco use and alcohol abuse has well documented implications on healing.[31,32]

On discharge, recommendations are verbally reviewed with the patient and provided in written format with explanations for each to encourage compliance. Discharge recommendations include continuation of inpatient therapies to prevent deconditioning, pressure wounding, and discourage edema formation. The patient is discharged with an incentive spirometer to continue breathing exercises 10 times each hour while awake. Multimodal pain control is resumed and venous thromboembolism prophylaxis is uninterrupted. We maintain the strict elevation and bed rest protocol until pain and swelling is controlled. Once under control we recommend no more than 15 minutes of activity, per hour. It is recommended that the patient recreate our universal lower extremity elevation protocol to ensure proper elevation.[23]

Returning to home puts increased importance on ensuring their social support network is robust during the initial assessment. Close monitoring in the outpatient setting remains essential because uncontrollable pain is associated with soft tissue compromise and an enlarging hematoma necessitating the need to reassess for compartment syndrome.[4] We have found inspection of the soft tissues in the days preceding surgery to be beneficial to confirm appropriate timing of surgery and ability to safely return home following surgery; persistent swelling or worsening wounding heightens level of concern for compliance and/or ability to safely return home.

If outpatient cares are deemed appropriate, the recommendations provided for initial management are near identical to inpatient cares. The injured extremity is immobilized in a modified Sir Robert Jones dressing including the folded cotton padding and gauze "dressing sandwiches" with plaster posterior splint in slight equinus. Initial training for the patient to safely maintain non-weight-bearing status is provided with follow-up in physical therapy for further instruction. A multimodal pain regimen is initiated and recommended venous thromboembolism prophylaxis conveyed. Instructions on scheduled ice therapy and elevation are provided. The patient is seen in clinic within 24 to 48 hours for evaluation and initiation of further consultation if deemed appropriate. Written instructions and close follow-up cannot be undervalued in the outpatient setting.

Between initial evaluation and surgical intervention, timing should ideally not exceed 14 days to avoid initial coalescing of the comminuted fracture fragments and development of fibrotic stiffness to the soft tissues about the calcaneus.[2] Further delay is most commonly caused by inadequate soft tissue rebound secondary to lack of attention to ice, compression, and elevation therapy. If delay is necessary it is with known increased risk of complications.[2]

SUMMARY

Initial clinical management of closed DIACF necessitates appropriate management of the osseous and soft tissue components of the injury. Following a complete history of physical ruling out any other concurrent injuries, the primary goal is to perform a thorough lower extremity examination to determine if acute intervention is warranted. Once deemed stable, a baseline understanding of the complex nature of the fracture is established through plain radiographs and advanced imaging. Focus then turns to management with a protocol-driven approach for immobilization, elevation, ice, and pain control therapies. Final cares entail preparing the patient for the ensuing days and weeks by educating them of their injury, expected treatment course, and social/economic difficulties they will encounter. The initial clinical management of these life-altering injuries truly sets the stage of what is to come and what will be for their treatment course.

REFERENCES

1. Buddecke D, Mandracchia V. Calcaneal fractures. Clin Podiatr Med Surg 1999; 16:769–91.
2. Rammelt S, Zwipp H. Calcaneus fractures: facts, controversies and recent developments. Injury 2004;35:443–61.
3. Razik A, Harris M, Trompeter A. Calcaneal fractures: where are we now? Strategies Trauma Limb Reconstr 2018;13:1–11.
4. Sanders R. Displaced intra-articular fractures of the calcaneus. J Bone Joint Surg Am 2000;82:225–50.
5. Walters J, Gangopadhyay P, Malay D. Association of calcaneal and spinal fractures. J Foot Ankle Surg 2014;53:279–81.
6. Gardner M, Nork S, Barei D, et al. Secondary soft tissue compromise in tongue-type calcaneus fractures. J Orthop Trauma 2008;22:439–45.
7. Lawrence S. Open calcaneal fractures. Orthopedics 2004;27:737–41.
8. Gustilo R, Anderson J. Prevention of infection in the treatment of one thousand and twenty-five open fractures of long bones: retrospective and prospective analyses. J Bone Joint Surg Am 1976;58:453–8.
9. Park Y, Lee J, Hong J, et al. Predictors of compartment syndrome of the foot after fracture of the calcaneus. Bone Joint J 2018;100:303–8.
10. Rosenthal R, Tenenbaum S, Thein R, et al. Sequelae of underdiagnosed foot compartment syndrome after calcaneal fractures. J Foot Ankle Surg 2013;52: 158–61.
11. Bibbo C, Ehrlich D, Nguyen H, et al. Low wound complication rates for the lateral extensible approach for calcaneal ORIF when the lateral calcaneal artery is patent. Foot Ankle Int 2014;35:650–6.
12. Haddock N, Garfein E, Saadeh P, et al. The lower-extremity Allen test. J Reconstr Microsurg 2009;25:399–403.

13. Mahmoud K, Mekhaimar M, Alhammoud A. Prevalence of peroneal tendon instability in calcaneus fractures: a systematic review and meta-analysis. J Foot Ankle Surg 2018;57:572–8.
14. Strauss E, Petrucelli G, Bong M, et al. Blisters associated with lower-extremity fracture: results of a prospective treatment protocol. J Orthop Trauma 2006;20:618–22.
15. Schepers T, Ginai A, Mulder P, et al. Radiographic evaluation of calcaneal fractures: to measure or not to measure? Skeletal Radiol 2007;36:847–52.
16. Roll C, Schirmbeck J, Schreyer A, et al. How reliable are CT scans for the evaluation of calcaneal fractures? Arch Orthop Trauma Surg 2011;131:1397–403.
17. Roll C, Schirmbeck J, Müller F, et al. Value of 3-D reconstructions of CT scans for calcaneal fracture assessment. Foot Ankle Int 2016;37:1211–7.
18. Kapadia B, Elmallah R, Mont M. A randomized, clinical trial of preadmission chlorhexidine skin preparation for lower extremity total joint arthroplasty. J Arthroplasty 2016;31:2856–61.
19. Edmiston C, Leaper D. Should preoperative showering or cleansing with chlorhexidine gluconate (CHG) be part of the surgical care bundle to prevent surgical site infection? J Infect Prev 2017;18(6):311–4.
20. Schade V, Roukis T. Use of a surgical preparation and sterile dressing change during office visit treatment of chronic foot and ankle wounds decreases the incidence of infection and treatment costs. Foot Ankle Spec 2008;1:147–54.
21. Brodell J, Axon D, Evarts C. The Robert Jones bandage. J Bone Joint Surg Br 1986;68:776–9.
22. Elliott A, Roukis T. Anterior incision offloading for primary and revision total ankle replacement: a comparative analysis of two techniques. Open Orthop J 2017;11:678–86.
23. Schweinberger M, Roukis T. Effectiveness of instituting a specific bed protocol in reducing complications associated with bed rest. J Foot Ankle Surg 2010;43:340–7.
24. Deal D, Tipton J, Rosencrance E, et al. Ice reduces edema. J Bone Joint Surg Am 2002;84:1573–8.
25. Kohring J, Orgain N. Multimodal analgesia in foot and ankle surgery. Orthop Clin North Am 2017;48:495–505.
26. Williams J, Little M, Kramer P, et al. Incidence of preoperative deep vein thrombosis in calcaneal fractures. J Orthop Trauma 2016;30:242–5.
27. Knudson M, Ikossi D, Khaw L, et al. Thromboembolism after trauma. Ann Surg 2004;240:490–8.
28. Wells P. Use of a clinical model for safe management of patients with suspected pulmonary embolism. Ann Intern Med 1998;129:997.
29. Modi S, Deisler R, Gozel K, et al. Wells criteria for DVT is a reliable clinical tool to assess the risk of deep venous thrombosis in trauma patients. World J Emerg Surg 2016;11:24.
30. Fleischer A, Abicht B, Baker J, et al. American College of Foot and Ankle Surgeons' Clinical Consensus Statement: risk, prevention and diagnosis of venous thromboembolism disease in foot and ankle surgery and injuries requiring immobilization. J Foot Ankle Surg 2015;54:497–507.
31. Chakkalakal D. Alcohol-induced bone loss and deficient bone repair. Alcohol Clin Exp Res 2005;29:2077–90.
32. Truntzer J, Vopat B, Feldstein M, et al. Smoking cessation and bone healing: optimal cessation timing. Eur J Orthop Surg Traumatol 2014;25:211–5.

Surgical Management of Displaced Intra-Articular Calcaneal Fractures

What Matters Most?

George T. Liu, DPM*, Michael D. Vanpelt, DPM, Trapper Lalli, MD,
Katherine M. Raspovic, DPM, Dane K. Wukich, MD

KEYWORDS

- Intra-articular fracture • Calcaneal fracture • Functional outcomes
- Wound complications

KEY POINTS

- Anatomic reduction of the posterior facet of the subtalar joint of displaced intra-articular calcaneal fractures is associated with improved functional outcomes.
- Restoring Böhler angle is associated with improved functional outcomes.
- Severity of pretreatment Böhler angle and Sanders classification are prognostic of poor outcomes.
- Minimally invasive reduction and fixation techniques reduce complications of infection and wound dehiscence.
- Adequate institutional volume and experience reduce infections, complications, and need for early subtalar arthrodesis.

INTRODUCTION

Fractures of the calcaneus are severe and complex injuries that result from a fall from height or motor vehicle accident and occur with an annual incidence of 11.5 per 100,000 person-years.[1] Fractures of the calcaneus comprise 1.2% of fractures in the human body and 62.4% of all tarsal bone fractures in the foot.[2] Approximately two-thirds of all calcaneal fractures involve the articular facet.[1]

The health-related quality of life of patients who suffer from displaced intra-articular fractures of the calcaneus is generally poor. Functional outcomes are lower compared

Disclosures: The authors have no conflicts of financial interest related to the contents of this article.
Department of Orthopaedic Surgery, University of Texas Southwestern Medical Center, 1801 Inwood Road, Dallas, TX 75390-8883, USA
* Corresponding author.
E-mail address: George.liu@utsouthwestern.edu

with patients who undergo open reduction internal fixation (ORIF) for tarsometatarsal fractures and malleolar fractures, but fare better than tibial fractures that involve the plafond.[3–6]

In general, patients who sustain calcaneal fractures report a lower health-related quality of life than patients who suffer from chronic disability or chronic medical illnesses.[5,7] Less than 25% of patients with a displaced intra-articular calcaneal fracture (DIACF) are able to return to the same line of work.[8]

Treated nonoperatively, patients develop posttraumatic arthritis, chronic heel deformity, and malalignment of the mechanical axis of the limb.[9,10]

The decision to treat displaced fractures operatively versus nonoperatively is controversial. Several prospective randomized controlled trials (RCTs) with long-term follow-up demonstrated no difference in functional outcomes between operatively and nonoperatively treated calcaneal fractures.[11–13] However, patients who are treated nonoperatively are nearly 6 times more likely to require distraction subtalar joint arthrodesis,[14] whereas patients who undergo ORIF for DIACFs have a 41% relative risk reduction of posttraumatic arthritis.[12] Subgroup and post hoc analysis of these studies identified certain fracture patterns that are associated with improved functional outcomes after ORIF.[11,12,15] Anatomic articular reduction, restoration of Böhler angle, female gender, younger patients, patients with lighter workload, non-Worker's compensation, and lower-grade Sanders classification had improved functional outcome scores with operative compared with nonoperative management.

ARTICULAR REDUCTION

The biomechanical function of the subtalar joint is complex, permitting high axial loads to be transferred from the leg to the foot. In addition to vertical load, the subtalar joint permits motion in the coronal plane. The subtalar joint consists of the anterior, middle, and posterior facet and motion and has a helical movement with axis of movement oriented inclination of 42° in the sagittal plane and 23° medially in the axial plane.[16,17] Clinically, the motion of the subtalar joint is translated into approximately 20° of inversion and 10° eversion of the heel.[17] On heel strike of the gait phase, the subtalar joint everts to dissipate the initial ground reactive forces.

Nonanatomic reduction of the subtalar joint may result in incongruent articular contact leading to abnormal focal distribution of contact pressures, which accelerates joint degeneration.[18,19] In addition, nonanatomic reduction restricts the ability of the subtalar joint to invert and evert, leading to difficulty in normal gait.

The quality of articular reduction of the posterior facet of the subtalar joint has been shown to be associated with improved clinical outcomes.[11,15,20–24] Buckley and colleagues[11] demonstrated the best clinical outcome scores were associated with anatomic reduction of the subtalar joint, with a trend for worsening outcome scores seen with ≥2 mm stepoff.

Rammelt and colleagues[25] used arthroscopy at the time of ORIF and found that improved functional outcomes scores were associated more anatomic restoration of the articular surface.

In their matched-cohort study of operatively treated calcaneal fractures in Worker's Compensation Board patients, Buckley and Meek[20] demonstrated that clinical outcomes scores improved with quality of articular reduction of the subtalar joint. Agren and colleagues[15] also reported that better clinical results were observed in patients with less than 2 mm of residual stepoff compared with patients with greater than 2 mm in an 8- to 12-year follow-up study.

BÖHLER ANGLE

Lorenz Böhler first described a "tuber-joint angle" formed by the intersection between a line from the anterior process of the calcaneus to the superior portion the posterior facet of the subtalar joint and that point to the superior portion of the calcaneal tuberosity.[26] This angle, known as Böhler angle, normally measures 25° to 40° and is used as a radiographic measure for subtalar sagittal alignment and calcaneal height. A decreased or negative Böhler angle indicates flattening of the subtalar joint and loss of calcaneal height.

PRETREATMENT BÖHLER ANGLE

Preoperative Böhler angle has been used as an indicator of severity of injury and as a prognostic indicator for long-term functional outcomes. A lower Böhler angle is associated with a more severe injury pattern.[27] Su and colleagues[28] identified a significant correlation between lower preoperative Böhler angle and severity of Sanders classification. Csizy and colleagues found that a Böhler angle of less than 0° on initial presentation was 10 times more likely to require a subtalar joint arthrodesis compared with patients with angles greater than 15°. Loucks and Buckley[29] also reported the prognostic value of a severely depressed Bohler angle and strongly associated this with a poor 2-year clinical outcome regardless of treatment. They opined that a lower Böhler angle was more indicative of a higher energy pattern, resulting in trauma to both the bone and the soft tissues that contributed to the prognosis for poorer outcomes.

POSTOPERATIVE BÖHLER ANGLE

The prognostic value of Böhler angle for postoperative outcomes in displaced fractures is controversial. This controversy is largely due to the heterogeneity of studies and methodologic challenges with standardization of metrics used to evaluate clinical outcomes.

Three retrospective studies[30–32] and one 15-year follow-up of an RCT[33] demonstrated no correlation between postoperative Böhler angle and functional outcome at final follow-up. The prospective study of Louck and Buckley[29] suggested that postoperative Böhler angle had little prognostic value with either conservative or operative outcomes for DIACF.

Other studies demonstrate prognostic value of Böhler angle for postoperative outcomes in DIACF.[11,15,22,28,34–40] Paul and colleagues[22] in their mean 6.5-year follow-up of 70 cases of operatively treated DIACF demonstrated a satisfactory clinical outcome in patients with a postoperative Böhler angle greater than 10°. Makki and colleagues[40] in their report of mean follow-up of 10 years and 47 cases of operatively treated DIACF demonstrated a linear correlation between the American Orthopedic Foot and Ankle Society (AOFAS) hindfoot score and increased angle of restoration of Böhler angle (best outcome seen ≥30°). In their prospective RCT comparing outcomes between operative and nonoperative treatment of DIACFs, Buckley and colleagues[11] reported the best clinical outcomes in patients with posttreatment Böhler angles between 15° and 36° and the poorest outcomes with flat or negative Böhler angles between −56° and −1°. This trend was seen in both the operative and the nonoperative treatment groups. Another prospective RCT evaluating treatment outcomes of displaced fractures found that restoration of Böhler angle was more common in the superior compared with the inferior functioning group (mean, 17.6 vs 12.1; $P = .05$).[15] Su and colleagues[28] found that a more anatomic postoperative Böhler angle was significantly correlated with functional outcomes of operatively treated DIACFs, as seen in **Fig. 1**.

Accordingly, lack of restoration of Böhler angle was associated with poor functional outcomes.[11,15,35,41] Janzen and colleagues[35] reported severe functional impairment in patients with loss of subtalar joint range of motion and decreased Böhler angle. Paley and Hall[41] reported that a decreased Böhler angle ratio of the fractured to the uninjured contralateral side was a prognostic variable associated with an unsatisfactory outcome.

SANDERS CLASSIFICATION

The most widely used computed tomographic (CT) classification system of joint depression fractures of the calcaneus is the Sanders classification.[42] Sanders described 4 types of intra-articular fracture patterns based on coronal and axial cuts: type I consisted of nondisplaced fractures; type II involved 2-part fractures; type III was 3-part fractures; and type IV was ≥4-part or comminuted intra-articular fractures, as shown in **Fig. 2**.

In their series of 120 operatively treated DICAFs, Sanders and colleagues[42] reported on the prognostic value of the CT-based classification system. They found that the best outcomes were observed in patients with type II and III fractures, whereas the worst outcomes were seen in patients with type IV injuries.

A retrospective study of 127 patients by Rammelt and colleagues[43] found that the severity of intra-articular injury as defined by the Sanders classification correlated with worsening function.

Agren and colleagues[15] compared 28 patients who underwent operative treatment with 28 patients who were treated nonoperatively. Their 8- to 12-year follow-up study reported better functional outcomes in patients with Sanders type II as compared with type III fractures (odds ratio, 1.8; confidence interval, 0.6–5.1; $P = .16$). Patients with Sanders type IV fractures were 5.5 times more likely to require arthrodesis compared with Sanders type II.[14]

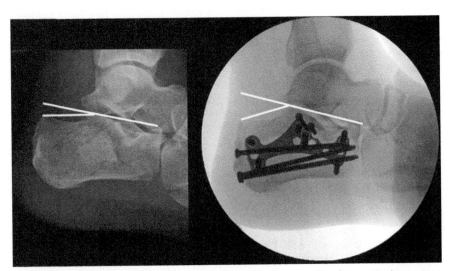

Fig. 1. Preoperative (*left*) and postoperative (*right*) imaging studies demonstrating restoration of Böhler angle.

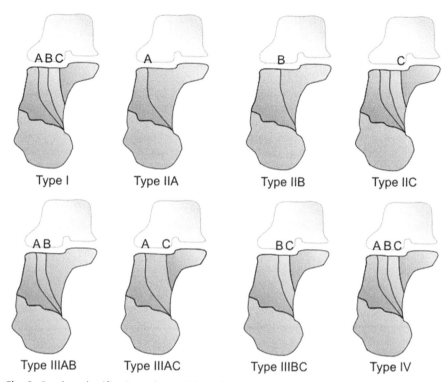

Fig. 2. Sanders classification scheme is based on a number denoting the number of intra-articular fragments and a letter indicating the location of the fracture or fractures.

A 10- to 20-year follow-up study by Sanders and colleagues[44] reported that type III fractures were 4 times more likely to require a fusion compared with type II fractures. Similarly, Buckley and colleagues[11] found that decreasing functional outcomes were associated with increasing Sanders classification. Patients with Sanders type II fractures were 2.74 times more likely to have Short Form-36 (SF-36) functional outcomes scores above the mean compared with patients with type IV fractures.

INSTITUTIONAL LOAD

Poeze and colleagues[45] performed a systematic review of 236 studies and 1656 calcaneal fractures evaluating the role of operative volume of DIACFs and associated complications. Institutions that performed less than one ORIF for a DIACF per month had a significantly higher median deep infection rate compared with institutions that perform more than one ORIF per month (8.9% and 1.8%, respectively). At this one ORIF per month cutoff, the odds for developing deep infection was 24. In addition, institutions that performed less than 0.75 ORIF of a DIACF per month were associated with a 6.4% increased rate of arthrodesis for subtalar arthritis than institutions that perform more with an arthrodesis rate of 1.9%. The study suggests that surgical volume and experience are associated with a reduction in the complication rate after ORIF.

OPERATIVE APPROACHES

The decision to perform a particular surgical approach is based on the need for exposure, surgeon experience, and reducing soft tissue complications (wound dehiscence and subsequent infection). Three approaches have been described, including the lateral extensile approach, sinus tarsi approach (STA), and the percutaneous approach.

Lateral Extensile Approach

The lateral extensile incision was originally described by Zwipp and colleagues[46] in 1989. This incision is "L" shaped with the vertical arm beginning approximately 1 cm anterior to the Achilles tendon and extends distally to the junction between the lateral skin and the glabrous plantar skin and then courses horizontally toward the base of the fifth metatarsal. The fasciocutaneous flap is raised in a full-thickness fashion, and "no-touch technique" retraction is often used to minimize trauma to the tissue flap. The approach provides optimal exposure of the lateral wall of the calcaneus, posterior facet of the subtalar joint, and the calcaneocuboid joint to allow reduction of both the intra-articular and the periarticular components of the calcaneal fracture, as seen in **Fig. 3**. Despite efforts to protect the lateral calcaneal flap, wound-related complications are prevalent. In 1999, Borrelli and Lashgari[47] performed a cadaveric study of the arterial supply to the lateral calcaneal flap of the hindfoot and found that the lateral calcaneal branch of the peroneal artery was also supplied by the lateral malleolar artery and the lateral tarsal artery. They found that the lateral calcaneal artery provided arterial flow to the corner of the tissue flap when performing the lateral extensile approach, and it is at the highest risk for injury if the incision is placed in its proximity.

Sinus Tarsi Approach

Palmer[48] originally described his lateral STA for DIACFs in 1948. This approach allowed access of both the subtalar and the calcaneocuboid joints and anterior process of the calcaneus. This incision begins approximately 1 cm inferior to the lateral malleolus and extends distally toward the calcaneocuboid joint. Depending on the fracture pattern, this incision may allow for proper reduction with the benefit of a smaller incision and potentially decreasing the risk of wound complications (**Fig. 4**).

Percutaneous Approach

Percutaneous reduction and fixation of DIACF fractures are considered for patients without significant intra-articular involvement. Minimal invasive

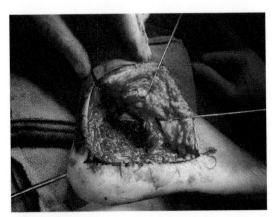

Fig. 3. Lateral extensile approach allows access of the subtalar joint, calcaneocuboid joint, and lateral wall of the calcaneus through lifting of the fasciocutaneous lateral calcaneal flap.

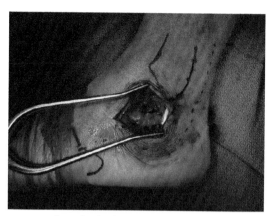

Fig. 4. STA allows access to the subtalar joint and anterior process of the calcaneus.

approaches can allow for adequate reduction and stabilization with percutaneous fixation (**Fig. 5**).

COMPARATIVE STUDIES OF SINUS TARSI AND PERCUTANEOUS VERSUS EXTENSILE LATERAL APPROACH
Wound Complications

Yao and colleagues[49] performed a meta-analysis of 2 RCTs[50,51] and 5 cohort studies[52–56] comparing the STA with the lateral extensile approach. In the pooled

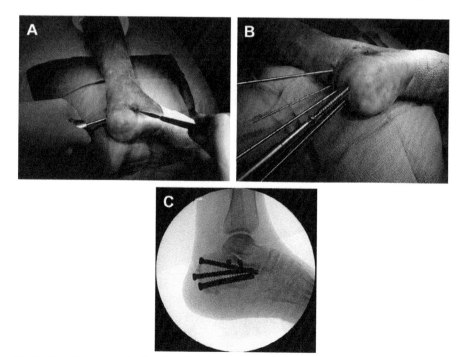

Fig. 5. Percutaneous reduction (A) and fixation (B, C) can be performed under intraoperative fluoroscopy through minimal incisional approaches.

analysis of the RCTs, a significantly lower incidence of wound complications was observed using the STA compared with the lateral extensile approach (0% vs 15.1%).[50,51] This lower incidence of wound complications after STA compared with lateral extensile approach was also reported in the cohort studies (2.7% vs 16.5%).[52–56]

Bai and colleagues[57] reported a meta-analysis of 4 RCTs[50,51,58,59] and 3 cohort studies[52,54,56] comparing STA versus lateral extensile approach for DIACFs. Significant difference with wound complications was seen in both the 4 RCTs (2.86% vs 19.23%)[50,51,58,59] and the 3 cohort studies (4.1% vs 21.21%).[52,54,56]

A meta-analysis of 8 studies by Zhang and colleagues[60] also reported lower wound-healing complication rates with STA at 2.63% compared with lateral extensile approach at 19.09%.

DeWall and colleagues[61] reported a retrospective comparison between 42 DIACFs that had percutaneous reduction and fixation and 83 DIACFs that had lateral extensile approach.

They reported a significant difference of deep infection between the percutaneous and lateral extensile approach group (14.3% vs 0%). In addition, wound complications occurred in 6.0% percutaneous group and 21.4% of the lateral extensile approach group.[61]

Böhler Angle

Although the principal concern is inadequate fracture reduction with limited fracture exposure through a STA, pooled analysis of the 2 RCTs demonstrated no significant difference when postoperative Böhler angle was identified.[50,51]

The mean Böhler angles were 25.89° for STA and 27.01° for lateral extensile approach, and the difference between the 2 groups was not significant.[60]

DeWall and colleagues[61] reported an average postoperative Bohler angle of 22.4° in the lateral extensile approach group and 25.3° in the percutaneous reduction group.

Functional Outcomes

Meta-analysis[57] of 2 RCTs[50,58] found no differences in treatment outcome in AOFAS outcomes scores between DIACFs treated with the STA versus lateral extensile approach.

In meta-analysis by Zhang and colleagues,[60] they reported no difference between excellent and good ratings seen between DIACFs treated with the STA versus lateral extensile approach. They also reported the mean visual analog score of 2.60 for STA and 3.91 for lateral extensile approach.[60]

Comparing percutaneous versus lateral extensile approach, there was no significant differences between the average SF-36 mental component summary score (48.6 vs 47.5) or physical component summary score (47.1 vs 39.6) between the 2 groups, respectively. In addition, no significant differences were seen between the Foot Function Index scores with 66.6 for the percutaneous and 70.7 for the lateral extensile approach group.

SUMMARY

DIACFs are complex high-energy injuries that can cause significant long-term functional impairment. Despite the controversies of whether these fractures should be treated operatively or nonoperatively, functional improvement can be seen with confounding variables that can be controlled by the surgeon. Anatomic reduction of the posterior facet of the subtalar joint and restoration of Böhler angle are associated with improved functional outcomes. The use of a minimally invasive approach in experienced hands may reduce the rate of soft tissue complications without compromising the quality of reduction. Adequate institutional surgical volume and experience of the surgeon are associated with a reduced rate of infections and less need for early subtalar arthrodesis.

REFERENCES

1. Mitchell MJ, McKinley JC, Robinson CM. The epidemiology of calcaneal fractures. Foot (Edinb) 2009;19(4):197–200.
2. Court-Brown CM, Caesar B. Epidemiology of adult fractures: a review. Injury 2006;37(8):691–7.
3. Obremskey WT, Dirschl DR, Crowther JD, et al. Change over time of SF-36 functional outcomes for operatively treated unstable ankle fractures. J Orthop Trauma 2002;16(1):30–3.
4. O'Connor PA, Yeap S, Noel J, et al. Lisfranc injuries: patient- and physician-based functional outcomes. Int Orthop 2003;27(2):98–102.
5. van Tetering EA, Buckley RE. Functional outcome (SF-36) of patients with displaced calcaneal fractures compared to SF-36 normative data. Foot Ankle Int 2004;25(10):733–8.
6. De-Las-Heras-Romero J, Lledo-Alvarez AM, Lizaur-Utrilla A, et al. Quality of life and prognostic factors after intra-articular tibial pilon fracture. Injury 2017; 48(6):1258–63.
7. Alexandridis G, Gunning AC, Leenen LP. Health-related quality of life in trauma patients who sustained a calcaneal fracture. Injury 2016;47(7):1586–91.
8. Veltman ES, Doornberg JN, Stufkens SA, et al. Long-term outcomes of 1,730 calcaneal fractures: systematic review of the literature. J Foot Ankle Surg 2013; 52(4):486–90.
9. Clare MP, Lee WE 3rd, Sanders RW. Intermediate to long-term results of a treatment protocol for calcaneal fracture malunions. J Bone Joint Surg Am 2005;87(5): 963–73.
10. Crosby LA, Fitzgibbons T. Intraarticular calcaneal fractures. Results of closed treatment. Clin Orthop Relat Res 1993;290:47–54.
11. Buckley R, Tough S, McCormack R, et al. Operative compared with nonoperative treatment of displaced intra-articular calcaneal fractures: a prospective, randomized, controlled multicenter trial. J Bone Joint Surg Am 2002;84-A(10): 1733–44.
12. Agren PH, Wretenberg P, Sayed-Noor AS. Operative versus nonoperative treatment of displaced intra-articular calcaneal fractures: a prospective, randomized, controlled multicenter trial. J Bone Joint Surg Am 2013;95(15):1351–7.
13. Griffin D, Parsons N, Shaw E, et al. Operative versus non-operative treatment for closed, displaced, intra-articular fractures of the calcaneus: randomised controlled trial. BMJ 2014;349:g4483.
14. Csizy M, Buckley R, Tough S, et al. Displaced intra-articular calcaneal fractures: variables predicting late subtalar fusion. J Orthop Trauma 2003;17(2):106–12.
15. Agren PH, Mukka S, Tullberg T, et al. Factors affecting long-term treatment results of displaced intraarticular calcaneal fractures: a post hoc analysis of a prospective, randomized, controlled multicenter trial. J Orthop Trauma 2014;28(10): 564–8.
16. Stiehl JB. Inmans's joints of the ankle. Philadephia: Lippincott Williams & Wilkins; 1991.

17. Sarrafian SK. Biomechanics of the subtalar joint complex. Clin Orthop Relat Res 1993;(290):17–26.

18. Bai B, Kummer FJ, Sala DA, et al. Effect of articular step-off and meniscectomy on joint alignment and contact pressures for fractures of the lateral tibial plateau. J Orthop Trauma 2001;15(2):101–6.

19. Brown TD, Anderson DD, Nepola JV, et al. Contact stress aberrations following imprecise reduction of simple tibial plateau fractures. J Orthop Res 1988;6(6): 851–62.

20. Buckley RE, Meek RN. Comparison of open versus closed reduction of intraarticular calcaneal fractures: a matched cohort in workmen. J Orthop Trauma 1992; 6(2):216–22.

21. Thordarson DB, Krieger LE. Operative vs. nonoperative treatment of intra-articular fractures of the calcaneus: a prospective randomized trial. Foot Ankle Int 1996;17(1):2–9.

22. Paul M, Peter R, Hoffmeyer P. Fractures of the calcaneum. A review of 70 patients. J Bone Joint Surg Br 2004;86(8):1142–5.

23. Basile A. Operative versus nonoperative treatment of displaced intra-articular calcaneal fractures in elderly patients. J Foot Ankle Surg 2010;49(1):25–32.

24. Gaskill T, Schweitzer K, Nunley J. Comparison of surgical outcomes of intra-articular calcaneal fractures by age. J Bone Joint Surg Am 2010;92(18):2884–9.

25. Rammelt S, Gavlik JM, Barthel S, et al. The value of subtalar arthroscopy in the management of intra-articular calcaneus fractures. Foot Ankle Int 2002;23(10): 906–16.

26. Böhler L. Diagnosis, pathology, and treatment of fractures of the os calcis. J Bone Joint Surg Am 1931;13:75–89.

27. Buckley RE, Tough S. Displaced intra-articular calcaneal fractures. J Am Acad Orthop Surg 2004;12(3):172–8.

28. Su Y, Chen W, Zhang T, et al. Bohler's angle's role in assessing the injury severity and functional outcome of internal fixation for displaced intra-articular calcaneal fractures: a retrospective study. BMC Surg 2013;13:40.

29. Loucks C, Buckley R. Bohler's angle: correlation with outcome in displaced intra-articular calcaneal fractures. J Orthop Trauma 1999;13(8):554–8.

30. Hutchinson F 3rd, Huebner MK. Treatment of os calcis fractures by open reduction and internal fixation. Foot Ankle Int 1994;15(5):225–32.

31. Kundel K, Funk E, Brutscher M, et al. Calcaneal fractures: operative versus nonoperative treatment. J Trauma 1996;41(5):839–45.

32. Mauffrey C, Klutts P, Seligson D. The use of circular fine wire frames for the treatment of displaced intra-articular calcaneal fractures. J Orthop Traumatol 2009; 10(1):9–15.

33. Ibrahim T, Rowsell M, Rennie W, et al. Displaced intra-articular calcaneal fractures: 15-year follow-up of a randomised controlled trial of conservative versus operative treatment. Injury 2007;38(7):848–55.

34. Parkes JC 2nd. The nonreductive treatment for fractures of the Os calcis. Orthop Clin North Am 1973;4(1):193–5.

35. Janzen DL, Connell DG, Munk PL, et al. Intraarticular fractures of the calcaneus: value of CT findings in determining prognosis. AJR Am J Roentgenol 1992; 158(6):1271–4.

36. Eastwood DM, Langkamer VG, Atkins RM. Intra-articular fractures of the calcaneum. Part II: open reduction and internal fixation by the extended lateral transcalcaneal approach. J Bone Joint Surg Br 1993;75(2):189–95.

37. Johnson EE, Gebhardt JS. Surgical management of calcaneal fractures using bilateral incisions and minimal internal fixation. Clin Orthop Relat Res 1993;(290):117–24.

38. Leung KS, Yuen KM, Chan WS. Operative treatment of displaced intra-articular fractures of the calcaneum. Medium-term results. J Bone Joint Surg Br 1993; 75(2):196–201.

39. O'Farrell DA, O'Byrne JM, McCabe JP, et al. Fractures of the os calcis: improved results with internal fixation. Injury 1993;24(4):263–5.

40. Makki D, Alnajjar HM, Walkay S, et al. Osteosynthesis of displaced intra-articular fractures of the calcaneum: a long-term review of 47 cases. J Bone Joint Surg Br 2010;92(5):693–700.

41. Paley D, Hall H. Intra-articular fractures of the calcaneus. A critical analysis of results and prognostic factors. J Bone Joint Surg Am 1993;75(3):342–54.

42. Sanders R, Fortin P, DiPasquale T, et al. Operative treatment in 120 displaced intraarticular calcaneal fractures. Results using a prognostic computed tomography scan classification. Clin Orthop Relat Res 1993;290:87–95.

43. Rammelt S, Zwipp H, Schneiders W, et al. Severity of injury predicts subsequent function in surgically treated displaced intraarticular calcaneal fractures. Clin Orthop Relat Res 2013;471(9):2885–98.

44. Sanders R, Vaupel ZM, Erdogan M, et al. Operative treatment of displaced intra-articular calcaneal fractures: long-term (10-20 Years) results in 108 fractures using a prognostic CT classification. J Orthop Trauma 2014;28(10):551–63.

45. Poeze M, Verbruggen JP, Brink PR. The relationship between the outcome of operatively treated calcaneal fractures and institutional fracture load. A systematic review of the literature. J Bone Joint Surg Am 2008;90(5):1013–21.

46. Zwipp H, Tscherne H, Wülker N, et al. Intra-articular fracture of the calcaneus. Classification, assessment and surgical procedures. Der Unfallchirurg 1989; 92(3):117–29.

47. Borrelli J Jr, Lashgari C. Vascularity of the lateral calcaneal flap: a cadaveric injection study. J Orthop Trauma 1999;13(2):73–7.

48. Palmer I. Mechanisms and treatment of fractures of the 08 calcis. J Bone Joint Surg 1948;30-A:2–8.

49. Yao H, Liang T, Xu Y, et al. Sinus tarsi approach versus extensile lateral approach for displaced intra-articular calcaneal fracture: a meta-analysis of current evidence base. J Orthop Surg Res 2017;12(1):43.

50. Basile A, Albo F, Via AG. Comparison between sinus tarsi approach and extensile lateral approach for treatment of closed displaced intra-articular calcaneal fractures: a multicenter prospective study. J Foot Ankle Surg 2016;55(3):513–21.

51. Xia S, Lu Y, Wang H, et al. Open reduction and internal fixation with conventional plate via L-shaped lateral approach versus internal fixation with percutaneous plate via a sinus tarsi approach for calcaneal fractures - a randomized controlled trial. Int J Surg 2014;12(5):475–80.

52. Kline AJ, Anderson RB, Davis WH, et al. Minimally invasive technique versus an extensile lateral approach for intra-articular calcaneal fractures. Foot Ankle Int 2013;34(6):773–80.

53. Takasaka M, Bittar CK, Mennucci FS, et al. Comparative study on three surgical techniques for intra-articular calcaneal fractures: open reduction with internal fixation using a plate, external fixation and minimally invasive surgery. Rev Bras Ortop 2016;51(3):254–60.

54. Weber M, Lehmann O, Sagesser D, et al. Limited open reduction and internal fixation of displaced intra-articular fractures of the calcaneum. J Bone Joint Surg Br 2008;90(12):1608–16.

55. Wu Z, Su Y, Chen W, et al. Functional outcome of displaced intra-articular calcaneal fractures: a comparison between open reduction/internal fixation and a minimally invasive approach featured an anatomical plate and compression bolts. J Trauma Acute Care Surg 2012;73(3):743–51.

56. Yeo JH, Cho HJ, Lee KB. Comparison of two surgical approaches for displaced intra-articular calcaneal fractures: sinus tarsi versus extensile lateral approach. BMC Musculoskelet Disord 2015;16:63.

57. Bai L, Hou YL, Lin GH, et al. Sinus tarsi approach (STA) versus extensile lateral approach (ELA) for treatment of closed displaced intra-articular calcaneal fractures (DIACF): a meta-analysis. Orthop Traumatol Surg Res 2018;104(2):239–44.

58. Li LH, Guo YZ, Wang H, et al. Less wound complications of a sinus tarsi approach compared to an extended lateral approach for the treatment of displaced intraarticular calcaneal fracture: a randomized clinical trial in 64 patients. Medicine (Baltimore) 2016;95(36):e4628.

59. Chen Z. Quantitative evaluation of postoperative effect of calcaneal frac-tures using Foot-scan system. Zhongguo Xiu Fu Chong Jian Wai Ke Za Zhi 2009;23:925–9.

60. Zhang F, Tian H, Li S, et al. Meta-analysis of two surgical approaches for calcaneal fractures: sinus tarsi versus extensile lateral approach. ANZ J Surg 2017;87(3):126–31.

61. DeWall M, Henderson CE, McKinley TO, et al. Percutaneous reduction and fixation of displaced intra-articular calcaneus fractures. J Orthop Trauma 2010;24(8):466–72.

Intra-Articular Calcaneal Fractures

A Literature Review of Atraumatic Incisional Considerations

Adam Landsman, DPM, PhD[a],*, Garrett Melick, DPM[b],
Anusha Pundu, DPM[b]

KEYWORDS

- Calcaneus • Fracture • Incisional approach • Wound closure

KEY POINTS

- Traditionally, the lateral extensile approach has been favored for intra-articular calcaneal fractures due to the high rate of anatomic restoration, but it is also associated with a high rate of wound disturbance.
- Incisional approach, timing of surgery, and wound closure techniques may all have an impact on postoperative outcomes for calcaneal fractures.
- The foot and ankle surgeon should consider vascular flow, or lack thereof, when designing the most atraumatic surgical plan for addressing intra-articular calcaneal fractures.
- Use of the Sanders classification may be helpful in guiding the decision for open versus minimally invasive techniques when treating intra-articular calcaneal fractures.
- Due to the fragile vascular supply of the lateral heel angiosome with traumatic injuries, low-tension closure techniques should be considered when treating calcaneal fractures through an open approach.

INTRODUCTION

Calcaneal fractures are a devastating injury that frequently results in the need for open reduction and internal fixation (ORIF). The structure of the calcaneus is often compared with that of an egg, with its relatively thin outer wall, and its propensity to break into many parts once cracked. Reconstruction of the calcaneus to anatomic alignment is crucial for restoring function to the foot, and minimizing pain, particularly

Disclosure: The authors have nothing to disclose.
[a] Division of Podiatric Surgery, Cambridge Health Alliance, Harvard Medical School, 1493 Cambridge Street, Cambridge, MA 02139, USA; [b] Cambridge Health Alliance, 1493 Cambridge Street, Cambridge, MA 02139, USA
* Corresponding author.
E-mail address: alandsman@cha.harvard.edu

Clin Podiatr Med Surg 36 (2019) 185–195
https://doi.org/10.1016/j.cpm.2018.10.014
0891-8422/19/© 2018 Elsevier Inc. All rights reserved.

podiatric.theclinics.com

in the subtalar joint region. Historically, the process of anatomic reduction and repair has involved ORIF, and relies on opening the soft tissue envelope to gain access to the bone.

Calcaneal fractures are frequently one component of a potentially more complex assortment of traumatic injuries. Depending on the type of trauma experienced, many times there is significant concomitant soft tissue destruction. Degloving and major lacerations introduce additional complications that will not be covered here. The more common scenario involves a calcaneal fracture from a high-impact injury, such as a fall from a ladder or a motor vehicle accident. In these cases, we anticipate fractures that involve joint depression, and fractures to the calcaneal wall. Oftentimes a tide mark, a blue stripe of ecchymosis along the plantar margin of the heel, and in some cases fracture blisters may appear. Standard convention dictates that ORIF surgery to the calcaneus is frequently delayed when possible until positive wrinkling of the lateral skin is observed and especially in the face of fracture blisters or excessive swelling, primarily due to the difficulties in closing the wound at the conclusion of this surgery. Delays of 1 or 2 weeks is not uncommon in these cases, to optimize the condition of the soft tissues.

When wound closure following repair of a calcaneal fracture is unsuccessful, this often leads to dehiscence and exposure of deep structures, including bone, deep fascia, and implanted hardware. Ultimately, this may lead to biofilm formation, cellulitis, osteomyelitis, painful scarring, and the need for additional surgery. In cases in which a wound has dehisced and internal fixation has to be removed before complete healing, the patient is much more likely to develop an uncorrected deformity and possibly decreased function, increased pain, and may ultimately require fusions or even amputation. Among cases involving trauma to the foot, calcaneal fractures have an unusually high level of wound complications. Carow and colleagues[1] pointed out that nearly 30% of patients having ORIF of the calcaneus will experience complications attributed to the wound. There has been much discussion as to why these wounds have a propensity for failure. Some of the factors considered can be found in **Box 1**.

Due to the inherent difficulty in successful treatment of dislocated intra-articular calcaneal fractures, it is critical for surgeons to take careful consideration in the preoperative planning stages. This requires careful attention to injury severity, risk factors for postoperative complications, and evaluation of the patient's soft tissue envelope. In this article, the authors focus on issues related to incision placement and the role of vascular supply in achieving wound healing with minimal complications with additional

---

Box 1
Causes for wound failure following calcaneus open reduction internal fixation

- Inappropriate soft tissue handling
- Patency of the lateral calcaneal branch of the peroneal artery
- Smoking
- Surgeon experience
- Diabetes mellitus
- Poor surgical timing in the presence of fracture blisters or excessive edema
- Infection
- Excessive dissection
- Wound closure technique

attention drawn to appropriate timing of surgical intervention and wound closure considerations.

INCISIONAL APPROACH CONSIDERATIONS

The lateral extensile incision remains the current standard of care for intra-articular calcaneal fractures, but it is associated with up to a 30% wound healing complication rate (**Fig. 1**). Proponents of its utility cite the importance of anatomic restoration of normal subtalar joint contact surfaces in calcaneal fractures,[2] and as such more experienced surgeons often favor the lateral extensile approach.[3] In a recent publication by Bibbo and colleagues,[4] their team evaluated the lateral extensile approach for calcaneal ORIF, and focused on the role of the lateral calcaneal artery in the instance of wound healing complications. They examined 90 consecutive intra-articular calcaneal fractures that were treated with traditional ORIF using plates and screws. Their sample consisted primarily of Sanders type 2 (37%) and type 3 (55%) fractures, with a few type 4 (8%) as well. In each case, the lateral calcaneal branch of the peroneal artery was assessed preoperatively by Doppler ultrasound, and wound complications were correlated with the quality of the preoperative vascular status. Of the 90 patients examined, 5 had non-Dopplerable signals in the lateral calcaneal branch. Overall, they observed 6 wound-related complications, with 5 of 6 being in the non-Dopplerable group. The complications in the non-Dopplerable group included 2 large nonhealing wounds and 3 wounds with complete dehiscence. In the one complication from a patient with a Dopplerable pulse, that patient developed a 2-cm dehiscence that went on to heal uneventfully. The difference in wound-related complications was statistically significant ($P<.0001$) among the group with a non-Dopplerable calcaneal branch from the peroneal artery. They also noted that among the patients who smoked (39% of the study population) and also had positive Doppler signals, only 1 of them developed a minor wound complication. Based on the significant increase in wound healing complications when the lateral calcaneal branch of the peroneal was non-Dopplerable, the authors recommended seeking out more minimally invasive alternatives that may afford preservation of the lateral heel angiosome.[4]

Carow and associates[1] also looked at the role of circulation as a potential factor in wound healing around the calcaneus. They evaluated 125 healthy subjects without history of rearfoot pathology or small vessel disease to measure oxygen

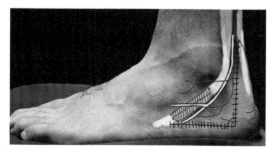

Fig. 1. The lateral extensile approach consists of a superior arm that begins 5 cm proximal to the lateral malleolus, with the incision bisecting the lateral malleolus and Achilles tendon and ending inferiorly at the level of the posterior calcaneal tuberosity. The inferior arm courses along the posterior edge of the heel toward the fifth metatarsal inferior to the level of the sural nerve, stopping just short of the fifth metatarsal base.

saturation and blood flow using a transcutaneous spectrophotometer in line with the location of a hypothetical lateral incision. They also considered cofactors, such as smoking history, gender, body mass index, age, and blood pressure. Flow was measured at depths of 2 and 8 mm. At the 2-mm depth, they found that flow was significantly higher along the course of a traditional Palmer and Ollier incision placement, as compared with the lateral extensile and extended lateral approaches (**Fig. 2**). Interestingly, however, the inferior aspect of the calcaneal tuberosity exhibited the highest blood flow and oxygen saturation when compared with other regions of the heel. Although the atraumatic nature of the study population makes it difficult to extrapolate conclusions to cases of traumatic calcaneal injuries, the investigators postulated that blood flow may not be the sole reason for wound healing complications at this region with typical lateral extensile approaches. In any case, this study demonstrates the variability in microcirculation across the lateral surface of the heel, which should be a major consideration when discussing incision placement.[1]

Despite the conception that open approaches offer higher rate of acceptable anatomic reduction, the increased rate of wound disturbance associated with open lateral techniques has garnered more attention toward different anatomic approaches and more minimally invasive approaches to calcaneal fracture surgical treatment. In 2000, Park and colleagues[5] published a retrospective review of 103 calcaneal fracture repairs via a limited Gallie posterolateral approach, in which a 3-inch linear incision is made along the lateral aspect of the Achilles tendon starting 1-cm proximal and posterior to the lateral malleolar tip and extending distally to the level of the calcaneus (**Fig. 3**A). They cited a low rate of wound complications and good functional outcomes with regard to subtalar joint mobility. Furthermore, they argue that this approach affords excellent visibility of the posterior facet while avoiding most pertinent neurovascular structures altogether.

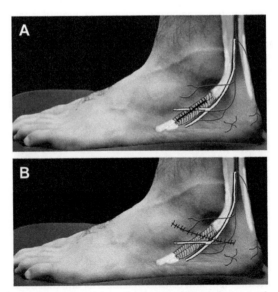

Fig. 2. (*A*) The Palmer approach consists of a 6-cm incision inferior to the lateral malleolus and parallel to the peroneal tendons. (*B*) The Ollier approach is an oblique incision starting 1 cm inferior to the lateral malleolus that extends distally and superiorly to the dorsolateral aspect of the talonavicular joint.

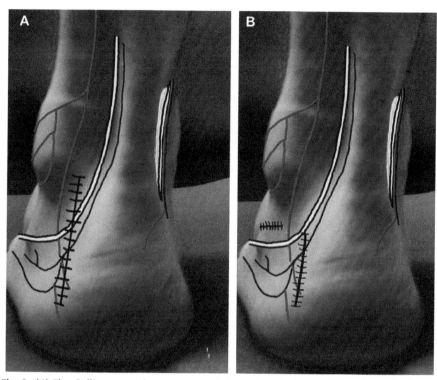

Fig. 3. (*A*) The Gallie approach consists of a 2.5-inch longitudinal incision along the lateral aspect of the Achilles beginning 1 cm proximal and posterior to the lateral malleolar tip down to the level of the calcaneus. (*B*) The Open Envelope consists of 2 longitudinal incisions. The first incision is a 6.5- to 7.0-cm full-thickness incision beginning 2.5 cm proximal to the lateral malleolus and courses lateral to the Achilles tendon. The second incision is a 1.5-cm linear incision of only skin over the anterior process of the calcaneus.

More recently, authors sought to describe a technique for posterior approach to displaced intra-articular calcaneal fractures via 2 longitudinal incisions (**Fig. 3**B).[6] The initial posterior incision is similar to that described by Park and colleagues[5] but the incision is extended slightly distally to encompass the superior arm of the traditional lateral extensile approach. The second incision involves a 1.5-cm longitudinal incision of only skin over the anterior process, with subsequent blunt dissection to place a calcaneal plate under the peroneal tendons. Among 42 fractures included, there were no deep infections and only 1 superficial pin tract infection at site of Kirschner wire (K-wire) placement. Similar to results published by Park and colleagues,[5] functional outcomes and radiographic parameters were noted to both be significantly improved. Use of the Sanders computed tomography classification[7] for operative approach considerations for displaced intra-articular calcaneal fractures is commonplace within the literature. For Sanders types II and III fractures of the calcaneus, previous literature remained equivocal regarding optimal approach. However, recent literature has provided important implications. Recently, a 2018 meta-analysis of randomized controlled trials was conducted to compare treatment of Sanders type II and III calcaneal fractures via lateral extensile and minimally invasive techniques (sinus tarsi and percutaneous approaches) (**Fig. 4**).[8] Among 8 studies meeting inclusion

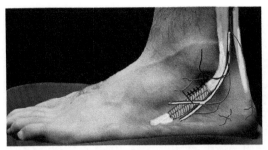

Fig. 4. The limited sinus tarsi approach consists of a 5-cm to 6-cm linear incision extending posteriorly from the anterior process over the lateral wall of the calcaneus.

criteria, all of the following outcome measures were improved in the minimally invasive treatment group for both grade II and III fractures: wound-related complication rate, visual analog scale score, time to surgery, and length of hospital stay. When statistical analysis of American Orthopedic Foot and Ankle Surgeons ankle-hindfoot scores was assessed for Sanders type II and III fractures specifically, increased functional outcomes were observed in the minimally invasive groups when compared with the lateral extensile group for grade II fractures only, with no statistical difference between the 2 groups in grade III fractures when pooled across studies. Also, no significant difference was noted in improvement of calcaneal width, length, Bohler angle, and Gissane angle between the 2 groups.[8] As a result, the authors of this study supported the use of minimally invasive approaches to prevent wound-related complications and afford similar or better subjective and functional outcome scores while providing similar anatomic reduction in Sanders type II and III fractures.

Similarly, in a multicenter retrospective review of 405 closed intra-articular calcaneal fractures treated via lateral extensile or minimally invasive (sinus tarsi approach or percutaneous approach), a statistically significant improvement in wound complication rate was noted in the minimally invasive group.[3] It is important to note that this study included Sanders fracture types I, II, III, and IV. Although wound complication rate was not increased according to fracture severity assessed by the Sanders classification in the lateral extensile group, there was a positive correlation of wound complication rate and fracture severity within the minimally invasive group.[3] As such, minimally invasive techniques were noted to provide decreased rate of wound complications, but more careful postoperative attention may be warranted for those undergoing this type of intervention in cases of more severe displacement and/or comminution.

With advantages of minimally invasive techniques previously demonstrated, it now becomes more important to evaluate the indications for small incisional approaches or percutaneous approaches in the treatment of intra-articular displaced calcaneal fractures. Multiple percutaneous systems are available, including a percutaneous cannulated screw fixation technique with calcium sulfate cement grafting,[9] a locked calcaneal nail inserted percutaneously,[10] and arthroscopically assisted percutaneous calcaneal osteosynthesis.[11]

Feng and colleagues[9] prospectively compared those treated via sinus tarsi approach versus percutaneous cannulated screw fixation with calcium sulfate cement grafting (which they had previously designed in 2006) in subjects with Sanders grade II and III calcaneal fractures. Among Sanders type II fractures treated with both techniques, anatomic reduction of the posterior facet was comparable, and wound complication rate was improved in the percutaneous group. For those with Sanders type III fractures, the results were more equivocal; posterior facet reduction was significantly improved in the sinus tarsi group, but wound-related complications remained favorable in the percutaneous group. Thus, it could be implied that minimally invasive percutaneous approaches are advantageous over the sinus tarsi group in type II fractures, but type III fractures may warrant more stringent evaluation of patient functional goals and risk for wound complications before deciding on an operative approach. Those with type III fractures and low risk for wound complication as well as high functional demand may benefit from the sinus tarsi approach, whereas those with higher risk for wound complications and/or lower functional demand may benefit from this percutaneous approach.

Arthroscopic assistance, while technically challenging, may be used in conjunction with calcaneal fracture repair. In cases of intra-articular derangement without significant orthopedic structural deformity, arthroscopic assistance through a percutaneous approach can offer the surgeon 2 important benefits: (1) limited incision and thus lower rates of wound-related complications, and (2) adequate evaluation of posterior facet step off and intraoperative restoration. In a study published by Schuberth and colleagues,[11] the senior surgeon describes initially performing percutaneous reduction of the tuberosity fragment to the sustentacular fragment followed by superior mobilization and temporary K-wire fixation of the depressed posterior facet fragment through a sinus tarsi stab incision. At this point, 1 of 2 approaches was used to visualize the reduction: (1) extension of the incision distally; or (2) introduction of a 4.0-mm arthroscope via sinus tarsi portals. In a retrospective analysis of 24 calcaneal fractures ranging from Sanders I to III treated via either of these approaches, these investigators found no instances of wound-related complications or subsequent subtalar joint fusion on average 2.8 years of follow-up. Also, they demonstrated statistically significant improvement in subtalar joint alignment with postoperative posterior facet step off of only 0.46 mm on average.

OPTIMAL TIMING OF SURGICAL INTERVENTION

Generally, it is accepted procedure to delay surgery until wrinkling of the lateral skin is observed, and most would also agree that significant high-energy trauma with fracture blisters or soft tissue compromise warrant delayed definitive treatment. However, given the large diversity in operative techniques and incisional approaches, the literature is quite variable in time to surgery based on incisional approach used. Thus, we feel it is pertinent to review the literature with regard to timing of surgical treatment in calcaneal fracture treatment.

Ho and colleagues[12] considered the postinjury timing of surgical repair via lateral extensile approach as a factor in predicting complications. They evaluated 53 patients undergoing ORIF with a lateral extensile approach, who were stratified into early treatment (32 fractures treated within 72 hours of injury), intermediate treatment (11 fractures treated between 72 hours and 10 days post injury), and delayed treatment (10 fractures treated >10 days post injury). Patients with open fracture, degloving injuries, neurovascular compromise, or immunodeficiencies were not included. Although there was no statistically significant data to support the impact of time to surgery on the complication rate, they did note that of all treatment groups, only 1 case of infection occurred and was found in the earliest treatment group. As previously discussed, the blood flow to the lateral heel angiosome is delicate and is dependent on the lateral calcaneal branch of the peroneal artery. Bibbo and colleagues[4] suggest that in those cases in which this branch is absent, the surgeon may want to consider delaying

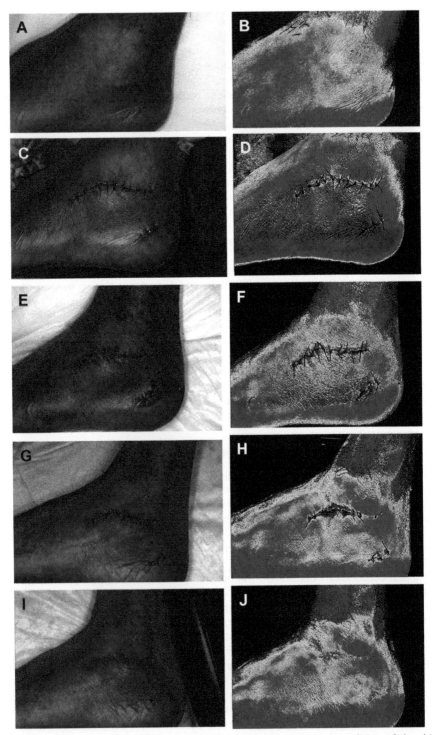

Fig. 5. (*A*) NIRS (http://www.kentimaging.com/) is used to assess the condition of the skin before surgery, immediately after surgery, and as the wound heals. This information can

surgery for a few weeks to allow for restoration of blood flow if planning ORIF via lateral extensile approach.

On the other hand, timing of surgery for minimally invasive techniques may follow a different set of principles. Kwon and colleagues[3] demonstrated an increased rate of wound complications when surgery was delayed at least 2 weeks after the injury compared with within 7 days of injury among those treated via sinus tarsi incisional approach or percutaneous approach. Conversely, similar to findings by Ho and colleagues,[12] they showed no statistical difference in wound complication rate according to timing of surgery among those treated via lateral extensile approach. As suggested by Kwon and colleagues,[3] minimally invasive approaches may afford a shorter time to surgery than more extensive incisional approaches. However, more research is warranted with respect to optimal timing according to specific incisional approaches used.

WOUND CLOSURE PRINCIPLES AND CONSIDERATIONS

Due to poor vascular viability, edema, and high rates of hematoma formation, incisional soft tissue flaps are at high risk of wound complications. As a result, most investigators recommend minimal soft tissue handling of incisional wound margins when proceeding with the lateral extensile approach. Compared with other foot and ankle surgeries, postoperative wound care is generally quite conservative. In their study, the standard postoperative protocol used by Bibbo and colleagues[4] involved placement of closed suction drains, bacitracin and iodophore gauze dressing, and both posterior and U plaster splints with use of antibiotics until drain removal. In addition, skin sutures and staples were not removed until 4 to 6 weeks postoperatively.

Wound closure of open approaches is normally performed in 2 layers, with various techniques used for superficial closure. In a study of various suture techniques in a single porcine model, it was determined that as tension was increased on the suture used, the Allgower-Donati modification of the vertical mattress technique[13] was associated with the smallest change in cutaneous blood flow when compared with vertical mattress, horizontal mattress, and simple interrupted suture techniques. Each of these other suture patterns exhibited no statistical difference when compared with each other at all tension increments.[14] As a result, the Allgower-Donati suture may be superior to these other superficial wound closure techniques with regard to preservation of blood flow. However, it is important to note that this porcine model involved only linear incisions, which is different from most operative approaches to calcaneal fractures. For this reason, a similar study assessing blood flow of different wound closure techniques specific to calcaneal fractures may provide important implications.

---

be used to assess the condition of the soft tissue envelope before surgery, and to monitor the perfusion of the wound and periwound areas after surgery. Preoperative image showing ecchymosis associated with calcaneal fracture. (*B*) NIRS image shows slight reduction in skin perfusion (*yellow areas*). (*C*) Immediate postoperative image showing a modified sinus tarsi surgical incision. (*D*) There is an increase in perfusion adjacent to the incision areas, consistent with an acute incision. Darker blackish areas are due to hematoma. (*E*) After one week, the wound continues to show signs of healing. (*F*) There is a corresponding subtle increase in perfusion of the periwound area with decrease in immediate inflammation. (*G*) Two weeks postoperative image. (*H*) Increased concentration of red areas adjacent to the incision line show an increase in perfusion posteriorly. However, the incision line itself shows some slight decrease in perfusion. (*I*) Three weeks postoperative image shows continued improvement and healing, without any sign of dehiscence. (*J*) Perfusion along the incision line has improved, and the wound has gone on to heal completely.

Despite the affirmed efficacy of negative pressure wound vacuum-assisted closure (VAC) to treat established wounds, the use of incisional wound VAC therapy to supplement closure techniques in lower extremity trauma is a relatively novel concept. In a multicenter prospective randomized controlled trial of 249 patients who sustained high-energy tibial plateau, tibial plafond, or calcaneal fractures, those in the treatment group had incisional wound VAC applied at (−)125 mm Hg continuous setting to supplement surgical incision closure.[15] Patients were kept in the hospital until documented minimal wound drainage (no more than 2 spots of drainage on gauze dressing of 2 cm or less over an 8-hour nursing shift) after negative pressure wound therapy application (NPWT), which was re-applied 2 days postoperatively and every 24 to 48 hours thereafter. NPWT was associated with decreased rate of wound dehiscence and associated infection compared with controls with regard to pooled high-energy lower extremity fractures. However, the investigators did not analyze each fracture type specifically.

ASSESSING TISSUE PERFUSION AND SKIN VIABILITY

Calcaneal fractures are frequently challenging to repair. The complicated nature of the fracture and difficulties in mobilizing the fragments into anatomic alignment is compounded by limited access resulting from a fragile soft tissue envelope. Previously, the issue of timing was discussed, as well as the importance of operating in the presence of only minimal soft tissue edema. Previous investigators have demonstrated the need for adequate microcirculation[1] and macrocirculation[4] at the time of surgery. Assessment of larger vessels, such as the lateral calcaneal artery, can include hand-held Doppler examination.

Light-based tools have been shown to be helpful in assessing the perfusion of the skin itself, to gage the potential for wound healing,[16] and can also be used to evaluate tension across the wound closure site. Near infrared spectroscopy (NIRS) (Kent Imaging, Calgary, AB, Canada) uses near infrared light to capture an image of a wound site by measuring the quantities of oxygenated and deoxygenated hemoglobin. The ratio of oxygenated to deoxygenated hemoglobin can be used as a measure of skin viability and perfusion. The following series of images demonstrate the level of tissue oxygenation before and after surgery (**Fig. 5**).

SUMMARY

When calcaneal fractures occur, the treating physician is faced with a large number of decisions that are required to bring about a good clinical outcome. From a surgical perspective, decisions have to be made regarding whether or not fixation is necessary, and if so, what will be used. Implicit in that thought process is the planning of the surgical approach. In this article, we attempted to show that there are numerous considerations including the level of edema, condition of the soft tissue envelope, posttrauma time, and circulation, both micro and macro. In our opinion, these factors should play a significant role in planning of the surgical incision, and may dictate the options available to the surgeon for repair.

REFERENCES

1. Carow JB, Carow J, Gueorguiev B, et al. Soft tissue micro-circulation in the healthy hindfoot: a cross-sectional study with focus on lateral surgical approaches to the calcaneus. Int Orthop 2018. Available at: https://doi.org/10.1007/s00264-018-4031-7. Accessed September 01, 2018.

2. Mulcahy DM, McCormack DM, Stephens MM. Intra-articular calcaneal fractures: effect of open reduction and internal fixation on the contact characteristics of the subtalar joint. Foot Ankle Int 1998;19:842–8.
3. Kwon JY, Guss D, Lin DE, et al. Effect of delay to definitive surgical fixation on wound complications in the treatment of closed, intra-articular calcaneal fractures. Foot Ankle Int 2015;36:508–17.
4. Bibbo C, Ehrlich DA, Nguyen HM, et al. Low wound complication rates for the lateral extensile approach for calcaneal ORIF when the lateral calcaneal artery is patent. Foot Ankle Int 2014;35:650–6.
5. Park I, Song K, Shin S, et al. Displaced intra-articular calcaneal fracture treated surgically with limited posterior incision. Foot Ankle Int 2000;21:195–205.
6. Prabhakar S, Dhillon MS, Khurana A, et al. The "open-envelope" approach: a limited open approach for calcaneal fracture fixation. Indian J Orthop 2018;52: 231–8.
7. Sanders R, Fortin P, DiPasquale T, et al. Operative treatment in 120 displaced intraarticular calcaneal fractures. Clin Orthop Relat Res 1993;290:87–95.
8. Zeng Z, Yuan L, Zheng S, et al. Minimally invasive versus extensile lateral approach for sanders type II and III calcaneal fractures: a meta-analysis of randomized controlled trials. Int J Surg 2018;50:146–53.
9. Feng Y, Shui X, Wang J, et al. Comparison of percutaneous cannulated screw fixation and calcium sulfate cement grafting versus minimally invasive sinus tarsi approach and plate fixation for displaced intra-articular calcaneal fractures: a prospective randomized controlled trial. BMC Musculoskelet Disord 2016;17:288.
10. Goldzak M, Mittlmeier T, Simon P. Locked nailing for the treatment of displaced articular fractures of the calcaneus: description of a new procedure with Calcanail®. Eur J Orthop Surg Traumatol 2012;22:345–9.
11. Schuberth JM, Cobb MD, Talarico RH. Minimally invasive arthroscopic-assisted reduction with percutaneous fixation in the management of intra-articular calcaneal fractures: a review of 24 cases. J Foot Ankle Surg 2009;48:315–22.
12. Ho CJ, Huang HT, Chen CH, et al. Open reduction and internal fixation of acute intra-articular displaced calcaneal fractures: a retrospective analysis of surgical timing and infection rates. Injury 2013;44:1007–10.
13. Mueller ME, Allgower M, Scheider R, et al. Manual of internal fixation. Techniques recommended by the AO-ASIF Group. 3rd edition. New York: Springer-Verlag; 1995.
14. Sagi HC, Papp S, DiPasquale T. The effect of suture pattern and tension on cutaneous blood flow as assessed by laser Doppler flowmetry in a pig model. J Orthop Trauma 2008;22:171–5.
15. Stannard JP, Volgas DA, McGwin G, et al. Incisional negative pressure wound therapy after high-risk lower extremity fractures. J Orthop Trauma 2012;26:37–42.
16. Landsman AS, Barnhart D, Sowa M. Near-infrared spectroscopy imaging for assessing skin and wound oxygen perfusion. Clin Podiatr Med Surg 2018;35: 343–55.

Closed Manipulation, Intraosseous Reduction, and Rigid Internal Fixation for Displaced Intra-Articular Calcaneal Fractures

Thomas S. Roukis, DPM, PhD

KEYWORDS

- CALCANAIL • Open reduction • Sanders classification • Surgery • Trauma

KEY POINTS

- Displaced intra-articular calcaneal fractures are life-altering events for those who sustain them.
- Controversy persists regarding the optimal surgical approach for management of displaced intra-articular calcaneal fractures; however, restoration of the calcaneal morphology and subtalar joint articular surfaces without inducing incision healing complications remains paramount for success.
- Minimally invasive techniques for the management of displaced intra-articular calcaneal fractures have become increasingly popular to reduce the known incision healing problems, but complete restoration remains difficult to reliably achieve.
- Closed manipulation of the calcaneus with a percutaneous caspar-type distraction device-assisted ligamentotaxis/tendinotaxis has fewer complications and more favorable functional outcomes compared with an open approach.
- The bone harvested from the posterior tuber of the calcaneus during creation of the working tunnel is an ample source of autogenous bone graft.

INTRODUCTION

Displaced intra-articular calcaneal fractures (DIACF) are life-changing events for most patients, resulting in some degree of permanent pain, swelling, and stiffness.[1] Surgeon experience does matter because centers performing less than 1 surgical repair of DIACF have a 5 times greater infection rate and 3.3 times greater subtalar

Financial Disclosure: Consultant for DePuy Synthes, FH ORTHO, Integra, and Novastep. Royalties received from CrossRoads Extremity, Novastep, and Stryker Orthopaedics.
Orthopaedic Center, Gundersen Health System, 1900 South Avenue, La Crosse, WI 54601, USA
E-mail address: tsroukis@gundersenhealth.org

arthrodesis rate than those centers performing more than one case per month.[2] Unfortunately, it is not practical to require surgeons managing DIACF to have an expert's knowledge, surgical expertise, and mastery of every treatment option available, including nonoperative management, open reduction with internal fixation, and knowledge of when to include bone grafting, percutaneous and minimally invasive reduction, and fixation methods, as well as primary subtalar arthrodesis techniques.[3,4] Although the optimal management of DIACF remains elusive, especially in those patients with bilateral involvement, treatment options should ideally be tailored to the fracture's unique personality and the individual patient-specific requirements. The dilemma exists about the long-term benefit of open primary operative intervention, even in experienced hands, given the high incidence of post-traumatic osteoarthritis, symptomatic hindfoot stiffness, retroperoneal tendon adhesions, wound dehiscence, and infection due to the extensive soft tissue trauma inherent with these injuries.[5] Although anatomic reduction of the articular surface of the subtalar joint is considered of significant importance, perfect anatomic reduction does not guarantee an improved clinical outcome due to the development of avascular necrosis of the periarticular fragments (**Fig. 1**).[2,4,5] Articular incongruity of 2 to 3 mm without step off has been demonstrated to be well

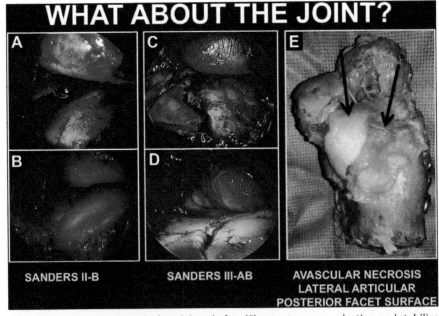

Fig. 1. Arthroscopic imaging before (A) and after (B) percutaneous reduction and stabilization of Sanders II-B fractures demonstrating near anatomic reduction of the articular surface of the posterior subtalar joint. Arthroscopic imaging before (C) and after (D) percutaneous reduction and stabilization of Sanders III-AB fractures demonstrating near anatomic reduction of the articular surface of the posterior subtalar joint. Despite reduction, as has been achieved, avascular necrosis of the lateral articular posterior facet surface frequently occurs as is demonstrated in this postmortem calcaneus managed with previous open reduction and internal fixation (E). The arrows point to the viable-appearing cartilage on the medial constant fragment and the adjacent absent remaining portion of the posterior subtalar facet.

tolerated by the subtalar joint.[6] Furthermore, restoration of normal calcaneal morphology, especially height,[7] has been demonstrated to restore normal kinematic and contact stress in the subtalar joint complex[8,9] as well as afford less complex secondary surgical intervention than a malunited calcaneus (**Fig. 2**).[10] What is clear is that incision breakdown with deep infection and sural nerve injury following open surgical approaches are devastating complications that cannot be easily resolved.[4,11] Ideally, management of DIACF will include preservation of vascular supply to all soft tissues and osseous fragments involved, use minimally invasive traction capable of restoring calcaneal morphology using ligamentotaxis/tendinotaxis along with indirect joint surface reduction techniques, afford delivery of minimally invasive but rigid internal fixation, and finally, allow for conversion to subtalar joint arthrodesis both during the index fracture management and for delayed salvage (**Fig. 3**).[12–17]

Recent literature supports the use of closed manipulation, percutaneous external fixation distractor-assisted ligamentotaxis/tendinotaxis to restore calcaneal morphology, intraosseous indirect subtalar joint surface reduction, and stabilization with a rigid, locked intramedullary nail contained within the calcaneus.[18–22] Representative implants that by and large incorporate these features include the CALCANAIL (FH Orthopedics, Chicago, IL, USA), C-NAIL (Medin, Nové Město na Moravě, Czech Republic), and VIRA Calcaneal System (Biomet Spain Orthopedics, SL, Valencia, Spain). Of these, the CALCANAIL is the only implant available in the United States for clinical use. In addition, the CALCANAIL is the only system that can be performed completely percutaneously or include a sinus tarsi

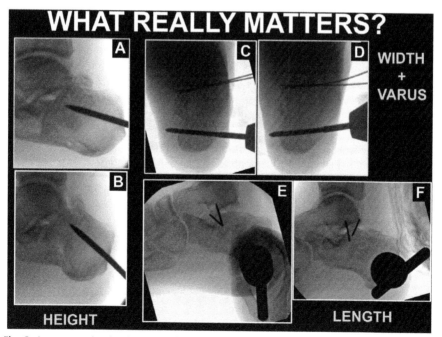

Fig. 2. Intraoperative image intensification views demonstrating restoration of the calcaneal height (*A, B*), width and varus reduction (*C, D*), and length (*E, F*). Restoring the calcaneal morphology is important to reduce stress and restore kinematics to the posterior subtalar joint as well as reduce complexity of future surgical interventions.

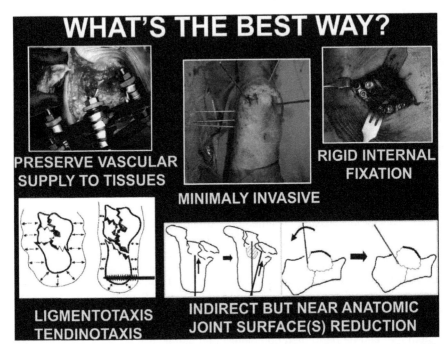

Fig. 3. The best operative approach for management of DIACFs includes preservation of the vascular supply to all involved tissues, ligamentotaxis/tendinotaxis, and indirect but near anatomic joint surface reduction and rigid internal fixation delivered through minimally invasive approaches.

incision for direct visualization of the subtalar joint reduction with primary fracture repair as well as be used to perform both a primary and a delayed subtalar joint arthrodesis.

LITERATURE REVIEW

One biomechanical cadaver dry bone study demonstrated the CALCANAIL is 3 times stiffer and has a significantly higher load to failure than a locked perimeter calcaneal plate.[23] Böhler angle was preserved in all CALCANAIL specimens, but in only half of the plated specimens included in this study. Another biomechanical fresh-frozen cadaver bone study demonstrated the CALCANAIL having no difference in load to failure, stiffness, or interfragmentary motion than a modern anatomic locked perimeter calcaneal plate.[24]

Simon and colleagues[19] conducted a prospective, nonrandomized clinical study of 69 DIACFs treated with the CALCANAIL. At a mean of 12.3 –month, 54 patients were evaluated due to 5 patients being lost to follow-up and 10 patients undergoing subtalar arthrodesis with the CALCANAIL fusion nail (6 primary and 4 secondary fusions). Böhler angle increased from a mean of 6.7° to 30.4° at 6 –month, and 84% had no intra-articular posterior facet step off based on computerized tomography scan performed at 3 months. No patient had malunion; ankle motion was preserved in 52 (96%) patients, and only 5 (9%) patients had less than 25% normal subtalar motion. Two patients developed sural nerve hypoesthesia that resolved spontaneously at 6 and 8 month. Six (11%) patients required hardware removal due to technical error, including 4 locking screws that were too long and 1 nail that was too long. Of note, no wound-healing problems or infections were encountered. At a mean follow-up of 12.3 months, 51 (94%) patients had a normal gait without a limp, 49 (91%) patients walked with mild or no difficulty, 45 (83%) patients had mild or no pain, and 37 (69%) patients reported no functional limitations. Similarly, Falis and Pyszel[20] conducted a prospective, nonrandomized clinical study of 18 DIACFs treated with the CALCANAIL at a mean follow-up of 12 months. Böhler angle increased from a mean of (−) 3° to 29° at final follow-up, and 89% had near or fully anatomic subtalar joint articular surface alignment based on postoperative computerized tomography scan. Two patients had implant-related problems, with one requiring removal of the implant. No nerve injury, wound-healing, or infection-related complications occurred. Mittlmeier and Herlyn[25] conducted a prospective, nonrandomized, matched-pairs study, of 40 consecutive displaced intra-articular Sanders classification 2 and 3 calcaneal fractures followed for 18 months postoperatively. There were 20 fractures treated with the CALCANAIL and 20 treated with a calcaneal perimeter plate and locking screw construct through an extensile lateral incision approach. Both groups achieved comparable restoration of the calcaneal morphology. The CALCANAIL demonstrated improved outcomes based on the American Orthopedic Foot and Ankle Society Hindfoot Scoring Scale and Foot Function Index Long Form. Postoperative computerized tomography demonstrated that the remaining subtalar joint articular defect was 0.7 mm for the CALCANAIL versus 1.6 mm for the perimeter plate and screw construct. No

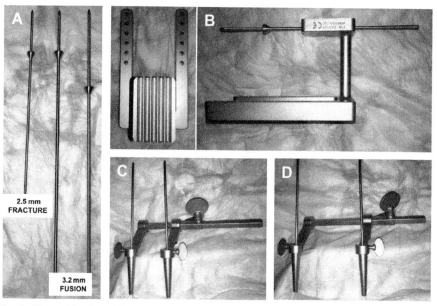

Fig. 4. The guidewire with stopper options available for, from left to right, calcaneal fracture repair, short and long options for subtalar joint arthrodesis (*A*). Note the difference in pin diameters. The positioning square demonstrating the available longitudinal tracts for the guidewire with stopper and available holes for the second wire (*B*). The caspartype distraction shown was placed over the Kirschner wires in the calcaneus and talus and secured with small thumbscrews (*C*). Turning the large thumbscrew distracts apart the guidewires and in turn the calcaneal fracture fragments (*D*).

wound-healing complications occurred in the CALCANAIL group, whereas 10% developed a wound requiring treatment in the perimeter plate and screw construct group. The investigators concluded that the CALCANAIL demonstrated improved functional outcomes, more anatomic reduction of the subtalar joint articular surfaces, and fewer complications compared with open reduction and internal fixation using a perimeter plate and screw construct through an extensile lateral incision approach.

SURGICAL TECHNIQUE

One should perform this procedure with the patient placed in the prone position under general anesthesia. Tourniquet control is not necessary. Under intraoperative C-arm image intensification, a guidewire with stopper is driven into the posterior tuberosity while maintaining alignment on the lateral view with the critical ankle of Gissane and on the axial view with the middle of the calcaneal tuberosity axis, which parallels any varus deformity present. A 3.2-mm Kirschner wire is placed bicortically through the positioning square perpendicular to the guidewire (**Fig. 4**A, B). A second 3.2-mm Kirschner wire is then placed bicortically into and perpendicular to the talar neck. The caspar-type distraction device is then placed over the Kirschner wires in the calcaneus and talus and secured with small thumbscrews (**Fig. 4**C). Next, the large thumbscrew is turned to gradually distract apart the calcaneal fracture fragments and open the subtalar joint until the calcaneal

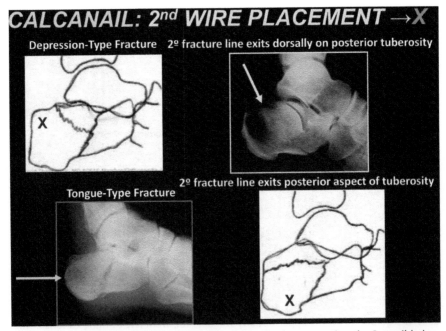

Fig. 5. Clinical drawings and representative radiographs demonstrating the 2 possible locations for the second guidewire placement (X). Specifically, the second guidewire should be placed in the superior aspect of the calcaneal tuber with joint depression-type fracture patterns where the secondary fracture line exists dorsally (*yellow arrow*) and the inferior aspect of the calcaneal tuber with tongue-type fracture patterns where the secondary fracture line exists posteriorly (*orange arrow*).

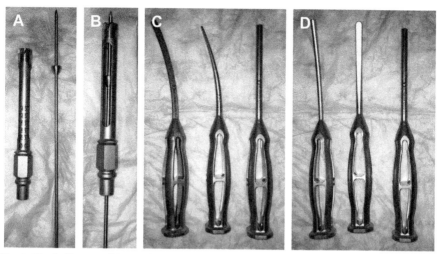

Fig. 6. The hollow trephine and guidewire with stopper separately (*A*) and as a unit (*B*). Side (*C*) and top (*D*) views of the curved, spatula-shaped, and straight bone tamps used to reduce the facture fragments.

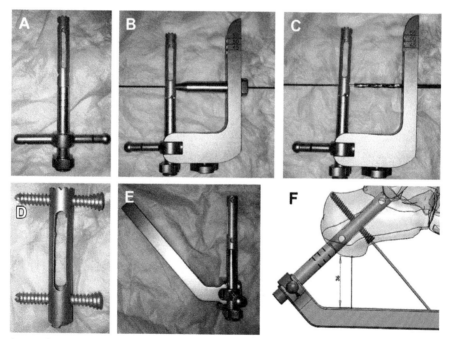

Fig. 7. The intramedullary locked nail attached to the T-shaped insertion handle with the rounded portion of the handle aligned with the D-shaped screw holes with the nail (*A*). The screw-targeting guide attached to the smooth lateral portion of the handle demonstrates placement of the smooth guidewire through the targeting sleeve (*B*). Once the targeting sleeve is removed, a cannulated drill can be used in dense bone to improve ease of screw insertion (*C*). The final intramedullary locked nail construct with 2 fully threaded screws and end cap inserted (*D*). The plantarly oriented aiming arm attached to the central portion of the T-shaped insertion handle (*E*). The plantarly oriented aiming arm with insertion of a fully threaded screw through the longitudinal slot in the intramedullary locked nail (*F*).

tuber has been brought out of varus as well as the length and height being restored (**Fig. 4**D). It should be noted that the location of the guidewire in the calcaneal tuberosity is dependent on the location of the secondary fracture line, as detailed in **Fig. 5**. A hollow trephine (**Fig. 6**A) is then placed over the guidewire (**Fig. 6**B) and advanced under image intensification to just beneath the subchondral bone of the posterior facet. The trephine is then removed, and the cylindrical bone graft contained within it is saved for later use. Next, the posterior facet fragments are sequentially reduced using the inferior surfaces of the talus as a template with a combination of curved, spatula-shaped, and straight tamps placed through the working chamber created by the trephine (**Fig. 6**C, D). Although dependent on the fracture pattern, most commonly the medial constant fragment is first elevated, followed by the lateral and then central fragments with C-arm image intensification used to track the reduction until the subtalar joint line is congruent. The length of the 10-mm-diameter fracture nail is measured with available lengths being 45, 50, and 55 mm and, once selected, the oblong window is packed with the previously harvested autogenous bone graft from the trephine. The nail is then introduced through the working chamber (**Fig. 7**A) and locked with 2 bicortical cannulated, threaded locking screws placed through the alignment targeting device (**Fig. 7**B–D). A plantarly oriented aiming arm allows for placement of an

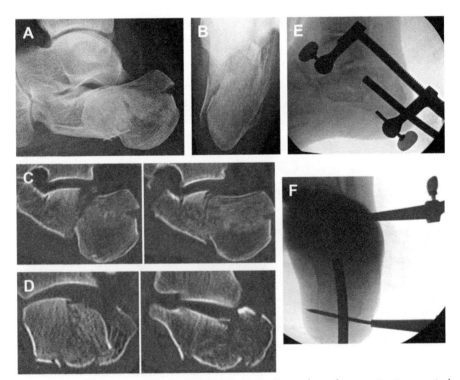

Fig. 8. Lateral (*A*) and axial (*B*) non-weight-bearing radiographs and noncontrast computed tomography lateral (*C*) and coronal (*D*) images of a DIACF in a 55-year-old malnourished male laborer who smokes tobacco and sustained a Worker's Compensation–related injury. Intraoperative lateral (*E*) and axial (*F*) image intensification views following caspar-type distractor-assisted restoration of the calcaneal morphology demonstrating intraosseous reduction of the articular segments of the posterior subtalar joint with a curved tamp.

optional oblique screw through the oblong window of the CALCANAIL to increase rotational stability and secure larger posterior calcaneal tuber fracture fragments (**Fig. 7**E, F). Independent screws placed outside the nail remains an option as well. Once the interlocking screws are placed, an end cap is inserted to facilitate removal if necessary, and then the distractor is removed. The patient is placed in a well-padded sterile dressing from toes to knee with the addition of a posterior splint to maintain the foot in slight plantarflexion to minimize pull of the Achilles tendon. Patients who are reliable remain in a dressing until skin incision has healed, which routinely occurs at the 2-week visit, followed by placement into a nonarticulated immobilization boot, and range of motion is initiated. Non-weight-bearing is maintained for 6 weeks followed by a gradual return to full weight-bearing and transition to shoe gear with serial surveillance radiographs obtained to assess osseous healing (see **Fig. 6**).

In the case of non-reconstructable damage to the posterior facet of the subtalar joint or late symptomatic posttraumatic degenerative disease, the same approach and instrumentation can be used to perform a primary arthrodesis of the subtalar joint with the 65-, 75-, or 85-mm-long 12-mm-diameter CALCANAIL with a minimally invasive sinus tarsi or posterior endoscopic approach used for joint preparation.

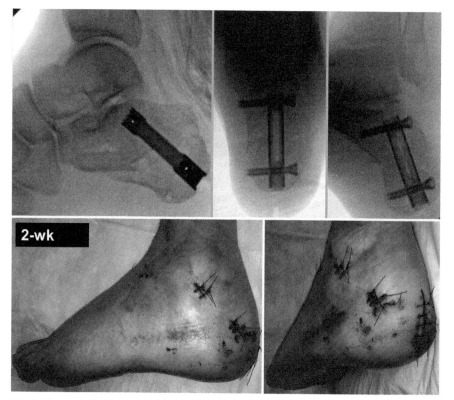

Fig. 9. Intraoperative lateral, axial, and Broden image intensification views (*top, left to right*) following final intramedullary locked nail insertion demonstrating maintenance of calcaneal morphology and near anatomic reduction of the posterior subtalar joint facet. Clinical photographs (*bottom*) at the 2-week follow-up visit demonstrating healed incisions despite the patient's ongoing tobacco use and persistent malnourishment.

COMPLICATIONS AND CONCERNS

Although the CALCANAIL offers several advantages over other forms of fixation, it is not without inherent limitations. A learning curve exists because the operative technique requires experience with percutaneous, minimally invasive, and open approaches to achieve consistent near anatomic reductions and incorporates maneuvers unfamiliar to most foot and ankle surgeons. The initial guidewire with stopper is placed freehand but must be carefully placed because all the subsequent steps are dependent on this wire. Heavy reliance on intraoperative image intensification, including repeated lateral, axial, and Broden views, can lengthen operative time, and the prone position can be disorienting for surgeons used to a lateral decubitus position. Even the inventor/consultant surgeons who were experienced with the device had patients with unacceptable joint reduction requiring secondary arthrodesis and technical errors resulting in the need for hardware removal.[18–20] Last, with surgical expenses under greater scrutiny, more literature is needed to better study the cost-benefit analysis of this device compared with contemporary fixation options in common use.

SUMMARY

Although soft tissue and osseous damage from the initial calcaneal fracture injury cannot be reversed, with minimally invasive reduction techniques and stout internal

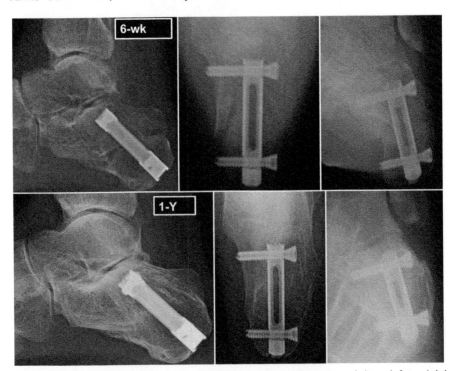

Fig. 10. Weight-bearing lateral, axial, and Broden radiographs at 6-week (*top, left to right*) and 1-year (*bottom, left to right*) follow-up of the same patient shown in **Figs. 8** and **9** demonstrating progressive osseous healing and maintenance of calcaneal morphology without any loss of correction. Note the near anatomic reduction of the posterior subtalar joint facet demonstrated on the axial and Broden views at 1-year postoperatively.

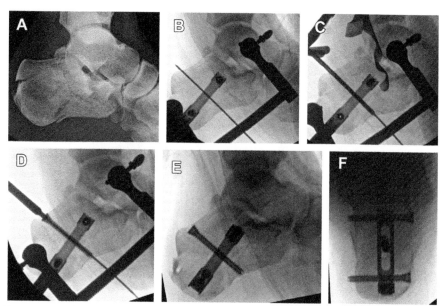

Fig. 11. Lateral non-weight-bearing radiograph (*A*) demonstrating a DIACF in a 42-year-old male roofer who smokes tobacco and sustained a Worker's Compensation–related injury. Intraoperative lateral image intensification view following insertion of the intramedullary locked nail and transverse locking screws demonstrating placement of the plantarly oriented aiming arm and guidewire delivered from the anterior-inferior aspect of the calcaneus through the posterior-superior aspect of the calcaneus (*B*). The cannulated drill is shown being performed from posterior-superior to anterior-inferior (*C*) that allows delivery of the fully threaded screw in the same direction (*D*). This approach allows for avoiding placement of the fully threaded screw through the delicate and vital plantar soft tissue structures but allows for secure capture of the osseous fragments and increases the rotational stability as noted on the final intraoperative lateral (*E*) and axial (*F*) image intensification views.

fixation the surgeon can limit further destruction and restore anatomic alignment as well as limit iatrogenic damage to the bone, articular cartilage, and soft tissue structures. Although not definitive, biomechanical cadaveric and prospective, nonrandomized, comparative clinical studies have demonstrated that percutaneous caspar-type distractor-assisted ligamentotaxis/tendinotaxis can reliably restore calcaneal morphology, achieve near anatomic intraosseous reduction of the calcaneal posterior facet fragments through indirect manipulation techniques, and deliver rigid internal fixation provided with a locked intramedullary CALCANAIL contained within the calcaneus. Highly comminuted DIACF of a wide variety of fracture patterns can be successfully managed as demonstrated (**Figs. 8–12**). Despite the need for more robust literature, the existing studies on the use of the CALCANAIL offer promising results, including no documented wound-healing problems or infectious complications, and may also allow for earlier operative intervention than other approaches. However, there is a clear need for noninventor/consultant surgeon prospective data to better assess outcomes of calcaneal fracture management with intraosseous reduction and internal locked nail fixation.

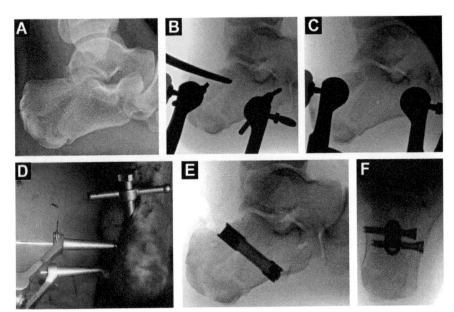

Fig. 12. Lateral non-weight-bearing radiograph of (*A*) a displaced intra-articular calcaneal beak-type fracture in a 34-year-old male firefighter who smokes tobacco and sustained a Worker's Compensation–related injury. Lateral intraoperative image intensification view demonstrating use of the caspar-type compression device to compress the fracture fragments together and the spatula-shaped bone tamp to manipulate the articular portion of the beak fracture (*B*). Lateral intraoperative image intensification view demonstrating anatomic reduction of the articular portion of the beak fracture and restoration of the calcaneal morphology (*C*). Intraoperative photograph of the posterior hindfoot demonstrating the percutaneous delivery of the intramedullary locked nail (*D*). Final lateral (*E*) and axial (*F*) intraoperative image intensification views following final intramedullary locked nail insertion demonstrating maintenance of calcaneal morphology and anatomic reduction of the posterior subtalar joint facet.

REFERENCES

1. Alexandridis G, Gunning AC, Leenen LP. Patient-reported health-related quality of life after a displaced intra-articular calcaneal fracture: a systematic review. World J Emerg Surg 2015;10:62.

2. Guerado E, Bertrand ML, Cano JR. Management of calcaneal fractures: what have we learnt over the years? Injury 2012;43:1640–50.

3. Sharr P, Mangupli MM, Winson IG, et al. Current management options for displaced intra-articular calcaneal fractures: non-operative, ORIF, minimally invasive reduction and fixation or primary ORIF and subtalar joint arthrodesis: a contemporary review. Foot Ankle Surg 2016;22:1–8.

4. Koutserimpas C, Magarakis G, Kastanis G. Complications of intra-articular calcaneal fractures in adults: Key points for diagnosis, prevention and treatment. Foot Ankle Spec 2016;9:534–42.

5. Eckstein C, Kottmann T, Füchmeier B, et al. Long-term results of surgically treated calcaneal fractures: an analysis with a minimum follow-up period of twenty-years. Int Orthop 2016;40:365–70.

6. Barrick B, Joyce D, Werner FW, et al. Effect of calcaneus fracture gap without step-off on stress distribution across the subtalar joint. Foot Ankle Int 2017;38:298–303.

7. Qiang M, Chen Y, Jia X, et al. Post-operative radiological predictors of satisfying outcomes occurring after intra-articular calcaneal fractures: a three dimensional CT quantitative evaluation. Int Orthop 2017;41:1945–51.

8. Yousri T, Wright SE, Atkins R. The effect of alterations of calcaneal height on the ankle and Chopart's joint: a cadaveric study. Clin Res Foot Ankle 2017;5: 242.

9. Xu C, Liu C, Li M, et al. A three-dimensional finite element analysis of displaced intra-articular calcaneal fractures. J Foot Ankle Surg 2017;56(2):319–26.

10. Radnay C, Claire M, Sanders R. Subtalar fusion after displaced intra-articular calcaneal fractures: does initial operative treatment matter? J Bone Joint Surg Am 2009;91:541–6.

11. Backes M, Schepers T, Beerekamp SH, et al. Wound infections following open reduction and internal fixation of calcaneal fractures with an extended lateral approach. Int Orthop 2014;38:767–73.

12. Zadravecz G, Szekeres P. Late results of our treatment method in calcaneus fractures. Aktuelle Traumatol 1984;14:218–26.

13. Forgon M. Closed reduction and percutaneous osteosynthesis: technique and results in 265 calcaneal fractures. In: Tscherne H, Schatzker J, editors. Major fractures of the pilon, the talus, and the calcaneus. New York: Springer-Verlag; 1993. p. 207–13.

14. Fröhlich P, Zakupszky Z, Csomor L. Erfahrungen mitder gedeckten Verschraubung intraartikulärer Fersenbeinbrüche Operationstechnik und klinische Ergebnisse. Unfallchirurg 1999;102:359–64.

15. Stulik J, Stehlik J, Rysavy M, et al. Minimally-invasive treatment of intra- articular fractures of the calcaneum. J Bone Joint Surg Br 2006;88:1634–41.

16. Schepers T, Schipper IB, Vogels LMM, et al. Percutaneous treatment of displaced intra-articular calcaneal fractures. J Orthop Sci 2007;12:22–7.

17. Schepers T, Patka P. Treatment of displaced intra-articular calcaneal fractures by ligamentotaxis: Current concepts' review. Arch Orthop Trauma Surg 2009;129: 1677–83.

18. Goldzak M, Mittlmeier T, Simon S. Locked nailing for the treatment of displaced articular fractures of the calcaneus: description of a new procedure with CALCA-NAIL. Eur J Orthop Surg Traumatol 2012;22:345–9.

19. Simon P, Goldzak M, Eschler A, et al. Reduction and internal fixation of displaced intra-articular calcaneal fractures with a locking nail: a prospective study of sixty-nine cases. Int Orthop 2015;39:2061–7.

20. Falis M, Pyszel K. Treatment of displaced intra-articular calcaneal fractures by intramedullary nail: preliminary report. Ortop Traumatol Rehab 2016;18: 141–7.

21. Pompach M, Carda M, Amlang M, et al. Treatment of calcaneal fractures with locking nail (C-NAIL). Oper Orthop Traumatol 2016;28:218–30.

22. López-Oliva F, Sánchez-Lorente T, Fuentes-Sanz A, et al. Primary fusion in worker's compensation intraarticular calcaneus fracture. Prospective study of 169 consecutive cases. Injury 2012;43(Suppl. 2):S73–8.

23. Goldzak MP, Simon P, Mittlmeier T, et al. Primary stability of an intramedullary calcaneal nail and an angular stable calcaneal plate in a biomechanical testing model of intraarticular calcaneal fracture. Injury 2014;45(Suppl. 1):S49–53.

24. Reinhardt S, Martin H, Ulmar B, et al. Interlocking nailing in intraarticular calcaneal fractures: a biomechanical study of two different interlocking nails vs. an interlocking plate. Foot Ankle Int 2016;37:891–7.

25. Mittlmeier T, Herlyn A. Calcaneal fracture fixation using a new interlocking nail reduces complications compared to standard locking plates. In: American Orthopaedic Foot and Ankle Society Annual Meeting, Seattle, Washington Proceedings. 2017. Available at: http://www.fhortho.com/wp-content/uploads/Calcanail_vs__Plate__Seattle__AOFAS_Poster_07_2017.pdf. Accessed November 27, 2018.

Sinus Tarsi Approach with Screws-Only Fixation for Displaced Intra-Articular Calcaneal Fractures

Tim Schepers, MD, PhD

KEYWORDS

• Calcaneus • Surgery • Sinus tarsi approach • Limited access • Less invasive

KEY POINTS

- Not all displaced intra-articular calcaneal fractures are manageable with the same treatment.
- Internal fixation should be tailored to the specific fracture characteristics and patient characteristics as well as the approach.
- Less comminuted fractures with sufficient bone stock are amenable to screws-only fixation.
- If, following screw-fixation, the construct is not stable enough to allow early motion, then a plate should be added.
- Future research should focus on the possible benefits of screw-only fixation versus plate fixation in the sinus tarsi approach.

INTRODUCTION

Of all foot injuries, fractures of the calcaneus have received the most attention in the literature. Throughout the years, practice has changed numerous times. Partially because not all displaced intra-articular calcaneal fractures (DIACF) are manageable with the same treatment, but even more so because of extended periods of rigid surgeon beliefs about how to treat DIACF best. The treatment spectrum ranges from nonoperative (early range-of-motion exercise) to operative. It is the latter that has given rise to countless procedures and modifications. There are 3 main surgical strategies: percutaneous (or minimally invasive), limited access (or less invasive), and the traditional extended open approach.[1] The benefits and downsides regarding reduction and complications per strategy are well known.

Disclosure Statement: The author declares there are no conflicts of interest.
Trauma Unit, Amsterdam UMC, Amsterdam Movement Sciences, Meibergdreef 9, Amsterdam 1105 AZ, The Netherlands
E-mail address: t.schepers@amc.nl

The sinus tarsi approach (STA) has regained interest in the last decade. It combines the benefits from both the percutaneous and the open approaches. The STA is an equally good reduction, but at a lower risk compared with the extended open approach.[2–4]

Following reduction, the fracture should be fixated to allow for early range-of-motion exercise and prevent collapse of the fracture. Various different ways of fixation are available, including external fixation, plate fixation, nail, Kirschner wires, and screws only.[5–9]

The current article deals with the STA in which the reduction is fixated using screws only. Indications and limitations, surgical technique, and possible pitfalls, as well as the available literature are discussed.

INDICATIONS

General indications for surgical treatment of DIACF are overall distortion of anatomy (height, width, and varus/valgus deformities) plus an incongruency at the subtalar joint. Subsequently, the goal of treatment should be an anatomically and biomechanically functional foot allowing for pain-free ambulation and the ability to wear shoes with limited adaptations.

Currently, in relation to operative versus nonoperative management, more meta-analysis than randomized trials exist, indicating that the dispute concerning which is better has not been settled yet.[10,11] All these randomized trials compare the extended lateral approach (ELA) to nonoperative treatment and show no conclusive evidence of superiority, which might indicate that the complications associated with the ELA outweigh the benefits of restoring the anatomy.[11] However, in the (sometimes inevitable) face of a possible secondary fusion, a previously restored calcaneus fares better than a more complex reconstructive procedure following a nonoperative management.[12] Albeit circumstantial evidence, a less complicated salvage procedure in the case of persistent complaints might be a good reason to opt for primary operative management.[11] In addition, the rate of secondary fusions following surgical repair is significantly lower than following nonoperative management.[13]

Historically the treatment of calcaneal fractures has been either nonoperative or minimally invasive.[14] In the early 1990s, the ELA became the "gold standard."[15,16] In that period, older less invasive techniques like the STA faded into the background.[9,17] It was not until 2 to 3 decades later that the STA fully reemerged.[2,18] As it appears, the pendulum is currently gradually swinging toward less invasive treatment of DIACF.[1]

The treatment of DIACF via a STA is a combination of open and percutaneous techniques. The subtalar joint is reduced open, and the reduction of the tuber (eg, the tongue-type [TT] fractures) resembles the techniques used in percutaneous techniques. Similarly, the fixation with a plate is an adaptation of the open technique, and the fixation using screws only is an implementation of percutaneous techniques. Several studies exist that compare the open (ELA) approach and subsequent plate fixation with percutaneous techniques and screw-only fixation.[19–22] Both techniques have been used in all types of intra-articular fractures; however, some have suggested that more complex fractures benefit from an open approach, such as the STA.[23]

More in detail to the indications of less invasive surgery with screws only fixation. The indications are mainly the less comminuted displaced, Sanders II and III, and DIACF. Substantial fragments are needed to fixate using screws only. More comminuted fractures are possible, but when one encounters insufficient stability, a plate must be added.

LIMITATIONS

Severely comminuted fractures, for example, Sanders IV fracture patterns, are less amendable to limited fixation, because stability is the key. Possible loss of reduction (see later discussion under "Pitfalls and Complications") may subsequently occur if fixation appeared insufficient. Loss of reduction may also occur in poorer bone quality (eg, osteoporosis). Preoperatively, stability should be tested following reduction and fixation. The screw-only fixation might be less suitable to correct widening. If, following restoring height and joint surface, and manual reduction with the aid of a broad periosteal elevator, widening is not corrected enough, a lateral plate might be added.

SURGICAL TECHNIQUE

The following is the preferred technique of the author.[5,6,24] Many variations have been described, which probably work equally well.

Positioning and Image Intensifier

The patient is positioned in a lateral decubitus position on a beanbag. A radiolucent table is used. The injured leg is flexed at the knee, and the contralateral leg is in neutral. The beanbag can be elevated at the level of the ankle in a way that the foot is free floating; this allows for inversion of the hindfoot during the procedure (**Fig. 1**).

A tourniquet is placed one hand width below the knee joint and is only inflated (to 100 mm Hg above the systolic blood pressure with a maximum level of 250 mm Hg) during the joint reconstruction and fixation part of the procedure.

The image intensifier is located at the opposite site of the table. With the foot slightly elevated in the horizontal plane, a lateral image can be obtained, when lifting the forefoot 45° and extending or flexing the ankle, a series of Brodéns views can be made. If one extends the leg and points the toes to the ceiling while tilting the C-arm, an axial view is provided (**Fig. 2**).

Anesthesia and Analgesics

General anesthesia is preferred for calcaneal procedures. Usually an ankle block is given by infiltrating all 5 nerves approximately 5 cm above the ankle joint.[25] In most patients, this ensures adequate pain relief immediately after surgery for the duration of about 12 hours, at which time the patient has reached adequate levels of oral pain medication. Alternatively, an ultrasound-guided popliteal block is provided by the anesthesiologist. As patients regularly go home the next day, a single shot block is commonly used.

Equipment

Besides the usually equipment for foot and ankle surgery, the following are regularly used:

- Small self-retaining retractor
- Kirschner wires in various widths (1.6 mm most often used)
- A small bone distractor
- 3.0-mm and 5.0-mm Schanz pin with T-handle
- 3.5-mm (non-)locking screws or 4.5-mm headless compression screws
- Periosteal elevator (2 sizes) and small Freer or Howard elevator
- Curettes
- 2.7-mm 30° arthroscope on occasion

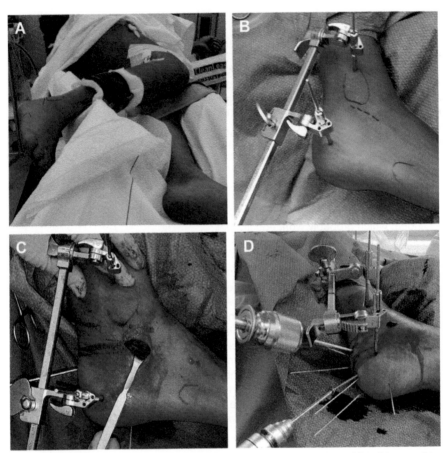

Fig. 1. Intraoperative positioning and approach. (*A*) Positioning in lateral decubitus position on beanbag. (*B*) Small bone distractor in place. (*C*) STA. (*D*) Varus correction with Schanz pin-and-screw fixation.

Surgical Procedure

An incision (STA) is made from 5 mm below the tip of the distal fibula toward the base of the fourth metatarsal (see **Fig. 1**). It is usually between 3 and 4 cm in length. The

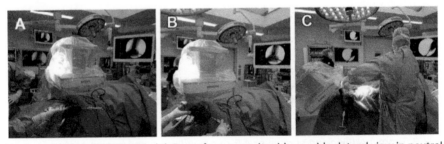

Fig. 2. Intraoperative imaging. (*A*) C-arm from opposite side provides lateral view in neutral position. (*B*) With lifting of the forefoot in various degrees of plantarflexion at the ankle, a Bröden view is created. (*C*) By extending the knee and rotating at the hip, an axial view is obtained.

peroneal tendons are protected and held plantar-ward. The sural nerve is not routinely explored, but if encountered, it is freed up and protected. The sinus tarsi is debrided to gain more access to the subtalar joint and to visualize the crucial angle of Gissane. Using a broad periosteal elevator and a small scalpel, the soft tissues and fractured lateral wall are separated. The peroneal tendon sheath is firmly attached (inferior fibular retinaculum) at the fibular trochlea of the calcaneus and requires some careful dissection to separate.

To gain more access to the subtalar joint, the small distractor or 5-mm Schanz pin is used. A small distractor with 2.5/3.0-mm half-pins is subsequently mounted from the talar neck or occasionally in the fibula (above the tibiotalar joint line) to the distal part of the tuberosity of the calcaneus. The pin placement is adjusted for any varus/valgus malalignment.

If the 5.0-mm Schanz pin is used, it is inserted from posterior, taking the varus deformity of the tuber into account. With a T-handle, the tuber is pulled outward (length), tilted to correct the axis, and pushed medially to correct the lateral displacement of the tuber. When the tuber and sustentaculum align, a 1.6-mm Kirschner wire is inserted on the medial side of the tuber into the sustentaculum.

After mounting the distractor, a small periosteal elevator is inserted via the STA into the fracture line to exit medially. The medial fragment is subsequently lifted and pushed against the talus. A 1.6-mm Kirschner wire is inserted from medial-plantar through the medial sustentaculum part of the fractured calcaneus and driven into the talus to create a constant/fixed part medially. By providing distraction, the tuberosity is brought downward, and space is created in the posterior talocalcaneal joint. When the fracture is older than 1 to 1.5 –weeks, the primary and secondary fracture lines sometimes need to be released with small osteotomes. When the tuber has been reduced adequately, it is fixated using Kirschner wires to the medial sustentaculum fragment. Alternatively, one could finish the joint reconstruction first if the tuberosity is kept at length using the small distractor.

Depending on the type of the intra-articular fracture (joint depression, JD; or TT), different reduction maneuvers are used. In case of a JD fracture with the use of a small bone rasp and a Kirschner wire in the lateral joint-fragment introduced through the STA as a joystick, the depressed fragments are lifted against the talus and fixated toward the medial constant fragment. Sometimes additional Kirschner wires from plantar are needed to stabilize these fragments before definitive fixation. In case of multiple intra-articular fracture lines, one works from medial toward lateral, reducing the lateral joint fragment last. This technique should restore the Böhler angle.

In case of a TT, a 3.0-mm half-pin (same as from the small distractor) is introduced from posterior to lever the fragment in place and is often aided with a small periosteal or Howard elevator via the STA. Reduction of the joint can be observed via the STA using image intensifier. Control radiographs with an intraoperative C-arm image intensification are made at various phases in the procedure.

At this stage, a decision is made whether joint reconstruction is feasible. In severe fractures, the option of a primary arthrodesis has been discussed with the patient preoperatively as part of the shared decision-making process. In case of a primary arthrodesis, the cartilage is removed from the subtalar joint; 2.0/2.5-mm drill holes are made on both sides, and two or three 7.3- to 7.5-mm cannulated screws are added to the fixation of the calcaneal fracture.

In comminuted fracture, caution is warranted with the large-diameter screws not to produce too much compression, because this will cause loss of height. A fully threaded positioning screw is subsequently used.

In Sanders III fracture patterns, one can fixate the middle joint fragment to the sustentaculum fragment using headless compression screws or using a Kirschner wire drilled through the medial skin of the foot. The joint reconstruction is finished using 3.5-mm screws in compression mode using a glide-hole or by using headless compression screws (3.0 mm or 4.5 mm).

Subsequently, the anterior process and Gissane angle are assessed. Following reduction of the posterior process first, Kirschner wire fixation is performed followed by one or 2 screws toward the sustentaculum. A bone substitute is rarely used to fill the neutral triangle cavity.

After joint reconstruction, the anterior process fragment or fragments are fixated toward the sustentaculum fragment. After this, the tuberosity is fixated toward both the anterior process fragment and the sustentaculum fragment using 2 or more screws (**Fig. 3**). One is inserted as medially as possible from the tuber into the sustentaculum. The second one is more horizontal in the lateral portion of the tuber into the anterior process, as close underneath the angle of Gissane as possible to further support the joint. An additional axial screw can be placed from the lateral tuber toward the lateral joint fragment.

Aftercare

Either a pressure bandage for 3 days or a negative pressure wound dressing is applied for 1 week (in high-risk wounds).[26] A plaster cast is not used routinely, and patients are

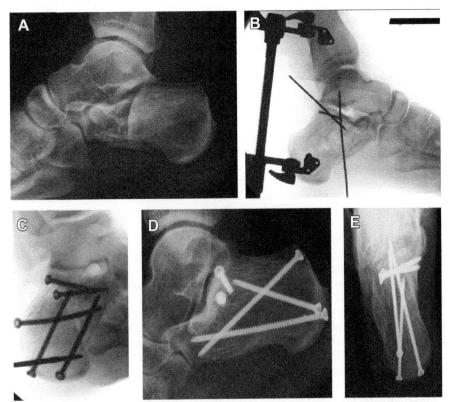

Fig. 3. Case example of 26-year old male patient with a TT fracture. (*A*) Preoperative lateral view. (*B*) Intraoperative lateral view. (*C*) Intraoperative Bröden view. (*D*) Postoperative lateral view. (*E*) Postoperative axial view.

allowed to exercise the ankle joint as soon as possible. Patients stay non-weight-bearing for 8 weeks, after which new radiographs (lateral, axial, and Brodén views) are obtained. In case of sufficient fracture healing, the patients are allowed to gradually increase weight-bearing. Often a schedule of "2 weeks–2 crutches" and "2 weeks–one crutch" is used. Patients are offered a referral for physical therapy should they feel the need.[27] They are well informed about the total recovery time of a displaced intra-articular calcaneal fracture, which may take up to 1.5 years.

TIPS AND PEARLS
Axial Locking Screws

One of the benefits of fewer implants should be a lower rate of implant removal. However, in some studies, the rate of implant removal has been reported similarly high as compared with the need for implant removal following plate fixation using the ELA.[28,29]

The need for implant removal might be lowered with the use of headless screws. However, these screws are typically designed to provide compression. This compression may affect the reduction that was obtained by distraction. In comminuted fractures especially, the use of compression screws may result in loss of reduction.

Alternatively, the author has found the use of locking screws beneficial for stabilization of the fracture fragments. The axial screws especially are used to fixate the tuber toward the sustentaculum and the anterior process, which often give rise to complaints of the bulky heads. The locking screw heads however sink into the cortex, lowering the risk of prominent implants, without giving compression between the fracture fragments (**Fig. 4**).

Primary Arthrodesis

The final functional outcome of DIACF is dependent on many different factors. Treatment (and expertise) and complications affect outcome. However, a large portion of outcome is dictated by the initial trauma. The "damage done" is irreversible. Several known factors related to the injury affect outcome negatively. These factors are fracture- and soft tissue–related factors. Less well known and substantially less investigated are the effects of patient characteristics on outcome.

The most well-known soft tissue condition known to reduce outcome is the open fracture. Fracture-related factors are severely comminuted fractures and fracture dislocations. These conditions lead to high rates of secondary arthrodesis, even following meticulous surgical reconstruction. One large series with long-term follow-up showed a nearly 50% secondary fusion rate in Sanders III fracture patterns.[30]

Depending on fracture, soft tissue, and several patient-related factors, the author preoperatively counsels patients about the option of a primary subtalar arthrodesis. If possible, a (near-) anatomic reconstruction is the goal. However, when chances of

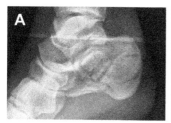
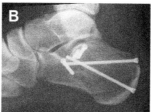
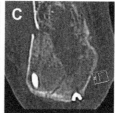

Fig. 4. Use of locking screws for axial stabilization. (*A*) Preoperative lateral view. (*B*) Postoperative lateral view. (*C*) Postoperative computerized tomography scan image.

a secondary arthrodesis in the future are high, then a primary arthrodesis is performed.[31]

The author uses the following fracture characteristics and patient characteristics to consider a primary fusion:

- Fracture characteristics: (1) a Sanders type III or IV; (2) fracture-dislocations; (3) initial Böhler angle less than 0; (4) open fracture; and (5) preoperatively noted extensive damage to the cartilage.
- Patient characteristics: (1) age >65 years; (2) lower physical demand; (3) doubts regarding compliance (ability of the patient to adhere to a non-weight-bearing regimen); (4) comorbidities (diabetes, smoking, obesity); or (5) at the request of the patient following the shared decision-making process.[5]

If 2 or more of these fracture and/or patient characteristics are present, the patient is counseled preoperatively to opt for a primary arthrodesis (**Fig. 5**).[5,32]

Currently at the author's hospital, about one-fifth of the operatively treated patients via an STA are a primary arthrodesis following restoration of height, width, and axis. A recent study comparing the ELA, STA, and primary arthrodesis showed a nonsignificantly higher outcome for the STA + reconstruction and no difference between ELA and STA + primary arthrodesis. The slightly higher outcome in the STA + reconstruction groups is likely biased attributed to "removing" and fusing the more severe fractures with expected poorer outcome.[5]

PITFALLS AND COMPLICATIONS

In calcaneal fracture surgery, "mistakes" are easily made. The main goals are restoration of overall anatomy and an as good as possible reduction of the subtalar joint. Besides failure in reduction, several other pitfalls exist that should be carefully dealt with peroperatively.

Stability and Osteoporosis

Screws-only fixation following reduction is an option, but should not be a means to an end. By this, the author means that screws only is one of the possibilities, but when preoperatively the stability appears to be less than desirable, then the option of a plate should be kept open.[33] Following incision and visualization of the subtalar joint, some distraction is provided. The subtalar joint fragments are reduced and temporarily fixated using Kirschner wires. Usually the subtalar joint is well stabilized using screws. The main problem lies in the neutral triangle. Following restoration of the subtalar joint, the tuberosity needs to be fixated. Fixation of the tuberosity is performed using one or more percutaneous screws from posterior. Subsequently, the subtalar joint should be tested. This can be done by inserting a Freer elevator in the subtalar joint and gently rotating it. If the subtalar joint and tuber move too much in relation to each other, then adding a plate is advised. An alternative method is by inverting and everting the heel or pronating and supinating the forefoot. The problem of residual instability plays a larger role in poorer bone stock.

Misplacement of Implants

Similar to in plate fixation of calcaneal fractures, choosing the correct length and position of the screws is a delicate process. Many articles exist on the proper techniques of screw insertion. These articles are mainly related to the correct placement of the sustentaculum tali screw, but are also in relation to the angled position of the calcaneocuboid joint and on the medial structures at risk.[34-40] Even though most of these

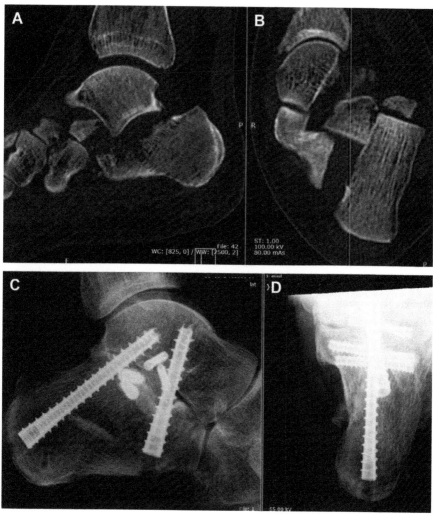

Fig. 5. Case example of 71-year old female patient with locked fracture dislocation of the calcaneus and lateral process fracture of the talus. (A) Preoperative sagittal computerized tomography scan image. (B) Preoperative semicoronal computerized tomography scan image. (C) Postoperative lateral view. (D) Postoperative axial view.

studies were designed for open surgical approaches, the principles are the same for less invasive procedures. Frequent checking under intraoperative C-arm image intensification in different planes or using preoperative 3-dimensional imaging may lower the need for postoperative revisions due to malposition of the implants.[34,41,42]

Insertion Percutaneous Screws

An additional, but rare, problem that can be encountered in inserting percutaneous screws is the epidermal inclusion cyst.[43] The stab incision used to insert the screw should be slightly larger than the screw head and should be gently opened up using a small hemostat. After insertion of the screw, the small wounds should be rinsed using a syringe with a large-bore intravenous cannula. If the incision is too small, then skin cells can be included in the wound where they can proliferate within the dermis. In approximately 200 cases in which axial percutaneous screws were inserted, 2 cases of epidermal inclusion cysts were encountered. In both cases, these had to be excised.

EVIDENCE FROM THE LITERATURE

Percutaneous techniques preceded the open techniques by several decades. The downside of the fully percutaneous techniques is the limitation in visualizing the posterior subtalar joint with intraoperative C-arm image intensification. Adding the STA has been a great step forward. Most studies in the literature focus on the difference in wound complications between less invasive procedures and extended open surgery. However, equally important are the stability of the construct (immediately and during follow-up) and the need for implant removal due to irritation.

Biomechanical (Stability)

In the study by Smerek and colleagues,[44] a Sanders type IIB fracture pattern was created in cadaveric feet and fixated using either a perimeter plate or percutaneous screws. No statistically significant difference was seen in load to failure and construct stiffness.

In 2010, Nelson and colleagues[45] investigated 2 fixation methods in cadaver calcanei. A nonlocking calcaneus plate was compared with a 4-screw configuration. A noncomminuted Sanders type IIB osteotomy was created. In this model, the screws-only technique provided similar or even better biomechanical stability.

Ni and colleagues[46] showed similar construct stiffness (stability) for Kirschner wire, cannulated screw, and plate fixation in a Sanders type III cadaveric model.

Finally, in case of osteoporosis and screw-only fixation, one could opt for adding (bone) cement. In a study by Rausch and colleagues,[47] this provided more stability than conventional fixed-angle locking plate osteosynthesis.

In conclusion, in relatively simple fracture patterns, without comminution, screws perform similar to plate fixation biomechanically. The calcaneal fracture models using osteotomies are of course not representative of daily practice in which fracture lines are not that well fitted and the central portion of the calcaneus is empty (neutral triangle) after pulling the posterior joint fragment out of the calcaneal body.

Clinical

The STA has proven equal to the ELA when looking at functional outcome independent of type of implant.[48–51] No studies were found that compared different fixation techniques following reduction via the STA. Kurozumi and colleagues[33] stated that in patients with severe lateral wall comminution and incomplete fixation of screws, additional plate fixation was performed. They mentioned the use of an additional plate in about 15% of cases.

Usually studies comparing screw versus plate fixation actually compared minimal invasive versus open techniques (either ELA or STA).[23,52] Feng and colleagues[23] compared minimal invasive (percutaneous) versus less invasive (STA). They found no significant difference in functional outcome for Sanders type II fracture patterns, and Sanders type III fracture patterns did better following the STA. However, this is more likely due to a difference in approach rather than a difference in fixation. Yeo and colleagues[50] compared the STA and the ELA, in which the STA received screw-only fixation. They found no difference in functional and radiological outcome, confirming the results of Kline and colleagues[20]

One of the areas future research should focus on is comparing less invasive plate (sinus tarsi plates) versus percutaneous screw fixation. This research should not only take complications and functional outcome into account but also construct stability and rates of implant removal of screw-only versus plate fixation.

SUMMARY

The less invasive STA is a huge step forward in the treatment of one of the oldest enigmas in foot and ankle trauma surgery. Not all calcaneal fractures are amendable to the same treatment modality; however, most can be restored adequately using this approach. Even though the late sequelae of arthrosis and the need for a secondary arthrodesis are not completely avoidable, an in situ fusion in a previously restored calcaneus, at the lowest possible risk, is a much easier procedure compared with a bone block distraction arthrodesis. The method of fixation is dependent on the fracture pattern (comminution) and the quality of the bone stock (osteoporosis). Screw-only fixation is a proven concept with similar results as plate fixation. In case of residual instability following screw-only fixation of a DIACF via an STA, a bailout by adding a plate might be considered to allow for early full range-of-motion exercise. Future research should focus on whether the possible benefits of screw-only fixation (less hardware removal, less wound complications) hold true.

REFERENCES

1. Sharr PJ, Mangupli MM, Winson IG, et al. Current management options for displaced intra-articular calcaneal fractures: non-operative, ORIF, minimally invasive reduction and fixation or primary ORIF and subtalar arthrodesis. A contemporary review. Foot Ankle Surg 2016;22(1):1–8.
2. Schepers T. The sinus tarsi approach in displaced intra-articular calcaneal fractures: a systematic review. Int Orthop 2011;35(5):697–703.
3. Schepers T. Towards uniformity in communication and a tailor-made treatment for displaced intra-articular calcaneal fractures. Int Orthop 2014;38(3):663–5.
4. Kwon JY, Guss D, Lin DE, et al. Effect of delay to definitive surgical fixation on wound complications in the treatment of closed, intra-articular calcaneus fractures. Foot Ankle Int 2015;36(5):508–17.
5. Dingemans SA, Meijer ST, Backes M, et al. Outcome following osteosynthesis or primary arthrodesis of calcaneal fractures: a cross-sectional cohort study. Injury 2017;48(10):2336–41.
6. Schepers T, Backes M, Dingemans SA, et al. Similar anatomical reduction and lower complication rates with the sinus tarsi approach compared with the extended lateral approach in displaced intra-articular calcaneal fractures. J Orthop Trauma 2017;31(6):293–8.
7. Takasaka M, Bittar CK, Mennucci FS, et al. Comparative study on three surgical techniques for intra-articular calcaneal fractures: open reduction with internal fixation using a plate, external fixation and minimally invasive surgery. Rev Bras Ortop 2016;51(3):254–60.
8. Zwipp H, Pasa L, Zilka L, et al. Introduction of a new locking nail for treatment of intraarticular calcaneal fractures. J Orthop Trauma 2016;30(3):e88–92.
9. Brattebo J, Molster AO, Wirsching J, et al. Fractures of the calcaneus: a retrospective study of 115 fractures. Int Orthop 1995;3(2):117–22.

10. Rammelt S, Sangeorzan BJ, Swords MP. Calcaneal fractures - should we or should we not operate? Indian J Orthop 2018;52(3):220–30.
11. Schepers T. Calcaneal fractures: looking beyond the meta-analyses. J Foot Ankle Surg 2016;55(4):897–8.
12. Radnay CS, Clare MP, Sanders RW. Subtalar fusion after displaced intra-articular calcaneal fractures: does initial operative treatment matter? J Bone Joint Surg Am 2009;91(3):541–6.
13. Buckley R, Tough S, McCormack R, et al. Operative compared with nonoperative treatment of displaced intra-articular calcaneal fractures: a prospective, randomized, controlled multicenter trial. J Bone Joint Surg Am 2002;84-A(10):1733–44.
14. Schepers T, Patka P. Treatment of displaced intra-articular calcaneal fractures by ligamentotaxis: current concepts' review. Arch Orthop Trauma Surg 2009; 129(12):1677–83.
15. Sanders R, Fortin P, DiPasquale T, et al. Operative treatment in 120 displaced intraarticular calcaneal fractures. Results using a prognostic computed tomography scan classification. Clin Orthop Relat Res 1993;290:87–95.
16. Zwipp H, Tscherne H, Thermann H, et al. Osteosynthesis of displaced intraarticular fractures of the calcaneus. Results in 123 cases. Clin Orthop Relat Res 1993; 290:76–86.
17. Soeur R, Remy R. Fractures of the calcaneus with displacement of the thalamic portion. J Bone Joint Surg Br 1975;57(4):413–21.
18. Ebraheim NA, Elgafy H, Sabry FF, et al. Sinus tarsi approach with trans-articular fixation for displaced intra-articular fractures of the calcaneus. Foot Ankle Int 2000;21(2):105–13.
19. Chen L, Zhang G, Hong J, et al. Comparison of percutaneous screw fixation and calcium sulfate cement grafting versus open treatment of displaced intra-articular calcaneal fractures. Foot Ankle Int 2011;32(10):979–85.
20. Kline AJ, Anderson RB, Davis WH, et al. Minimally invasive technique versus an extensile lateral approach for intra-articular calcaneal fractures. Foot Ankle Int 2013;34(6):773–80.
21. Kiewiet NJ, Sangeorzan BJ. Calcaneal fracture management: extensile lateral approach versus small incision technique. Foot Ankle Clin 2017;22(1):77–91.
22. Jin C, Weng D, Yang W, et al. Minimally invasive percutaneous osteosynthesis versus ORIF for Sanders type II and III calcaneal fractures: a prospective, randomized intervention trial. J Orthop Surg Res 2017;12(1):10.
23. Feng Y, Shui X, Wang J, et al. Comparison of percutaneous cannulated screw fixation and calcium sulfate cement grafting versus minimally invasive sinus tarsi approach and plate fixation for displaced intra-articular calcaneal fractures: a prospective randomized controlled trial. BMC Musculoskelet Disord 2016;17:288.
24. Schepers T. The sinus tarsi approach in displaced intra-articular calcaneal fracture. Expert Corner 2016. Available at: http://www.sicot.org/enewsletter-81-expert-corner.
25. Dingemans SA, de Ruiter KJ, Birnie MFN, et al. Comparable postoperative pain levels using 2 different nerve blocks in the operative treatment of displaced intra-articular calcaneal fractures. Foot Ankle Int 2017;38(12):1352–6.
26. Dingemans SA, Birnie MFN, Backes M, et al. Prophylactic negative pressure wound therapy after lower extremity fracture surgery: a pilot study. Int Orthop 2018;42(4):747–53.
27. Albin SR, Koppenhaver SL, Van Boerum DH, et al. Timing of initiating manual therapy and therapeutic exercises in the management of patients after hindfoot fractures: a randomized controlled trial. J Man Manip Ther 2018;26(3):147–56.

28. Backes M, Schep NW, Luitse JS, et al. Indications for implant removal following intra-articular calcaneal fractures and subsequent complications. Foot Ankle Int 2013;34(11):1521–5.

29. Tomesen T, Biert J, Frolke JP. Treatment of displaced intra-articular calcaneal fractures with closed reduction and percutaneous screw fixation. J Bone Joint Surg Am 2011;93(10):920–8.

30. Sanders R, Vaupel ZM, Erdogan M, et al. Operative treatment of displaced intra-articular calcaneal fractures: long-term (10-20 Years) results in 108 fractures using a prognostic CT classification. J Orthop Trauma 2014;28(10):551–63.

31. Buckley R, Leighton R, Sanders D, et al. Open reduction and internal fixation compared with ORIF and primary subtalar arthrodesis for treatment of Sanders type IV calcaneal fractures: a randomized multicenter trial. J Orthop Trauma 2014;28(10):577–83.

32. Schepers T. The primary arthrodesis for severely comminuted intra-articular fractures of the calcaneus: a systematic review. Foot Ankle Surg 2012;18(2):84–8.

33. Kurozumi T, Jinno Y, Sato T, et al. Open reduction for intra-articular calcaneal fractures: evaluation using computed tomography. Foot Ankle Int 2003;24(12):942–8.

34. Gitajn IL, Toussaint RJ, Kwon JY. Assessing accuracy of sustentaculum screw placement during calcaneal fixation. Foot Ankle Int 2013;34(2):282–6.

35. Lin PP, Roe S, Kay M, et al. Placement of screws in the sustentaculum tali. A calcaneal fracture model. Clin Orthop Relat Res 1998;(352):194–201.

36. Pang QJ, Yu X, Guo ZH. The sustentaculum tali screw fixation for the treatment of Sanders type II calcaneal fracture: a finite element analysis. Pak J Med Sci 2014; 30(5):1099–103.

37. Bussewitz BW, Hyer CF. Screw placement relative to the calcaneal fracture constant fragment: an anatomic study. J Foot Ankle Surg 2015;54(3):392–4.

38. Albert MJ, Waggoner SM, Smith JW. Internal fixation of calcaneus fractures: an anatomical study of structures at risk. J Orthop Trauma 1995;9(2):107–12.

39. Wang C, Huang D, Ma X, et al. Sustentacular screw placement with guidance during ORIF of calcaneal fracture: an anatomical specimen study. J Orthop Surg Res 2017;12(1):78.

40. Wang ZJ, Huang XL, Chu YC, et al. Applied anatomy of the calcaneocuboid articular surface for internal fixation of calcaneal fractures. Injury 2013;44(11): 1428–30.

41. Franke J, Wendl K, Suda AJ, et al. Intraoperative three-dimensional imaging in the treatment of calcaneal fractures. J Bone Joint Surg Am 2014;96(9):e72.

42. Janzen DL, Connell DG, Munk PL, et al. Intraarticular fractures of the calcaneus: value of CT findings in determining prognosis. AJR Am J Roentgenol 1992; 158(6):1271–4.

43. Posthuma JJ, de Ruiter KJ, de Jong VM, et al. Traumatic epidermal inclusion cyst after minimal invasive surgery of a displaced intra-articular calcaneal fracture: a case report. J Foot Ankle Surg 2018;57(6):1253–5.

44. Smerek JP, Kadakia A, Belkoff SM, et al. Percutaneous screw configuration versus perimeter plating of calcaneus fractures: a cadaver study. Foot Ankle Int 2008;29(9):931–5.

45. Nelson JD, McIff TE, Moodie PG, et al. Biomechanical stability of intramedullary technique for fixation of joint depressed calcaneus fracture. Foot Ankle Int 2010; 31(3):229–35.

46. Ni M, Mei J, Li K, et al. The primary stability of different implants for intra-articular calcaneal fractures: an in vitro study. Biomed Eng Online 2018;17(1):50.

47. Rausch S, Klos K, Wolf U, et al. A biomechanical comparison of fixed angle lock-ing compression plate osteosynthesis and cement augmented screw osteosyn-thesis in the management of intra articular calcaneal fractures. Int Orthop 2014;38(8):1705–10.
48. Li LH, Guo YZ, Wang H, et al. Less wound complications of a sinus tarsi approach compared to an extended lateral approach for the treatment of displaced intraar-ticular calcaneal fracture: a randomized clinical trial in 64 patients. Medicine (Bal-timore) 2016;95(36):e4628.
49. Sampath Kumar V, Marimuthu K, Subramani S, et al. Prospective randomized trial comparing open reduction and internal fixation with minimally invasive reduction and percutaneous fixation in managing displaced intra-articular calcaneal frac-tures. Int Orthop 2014;38(12):2505–12.
50. Yeo JH, Cho HJ, Lee KB. Comparison of two surgical approaches for displaced intra-articular calcaneal fractures: sinus tarsi versus extensile lateral approach. BMC Musculoskelet Disord 2015;16:63.
51. Zhou HC, Yu T, Ren HY, et al. Clinical comparison of extensile lateral approach and Sinus Tarsi approach combined with medial distraction technique for intra-articular calcaneal fractures. Orthop Surg 2017;9(1):77–85.
52. Fan B, Zhou X, Wei Z, et al. Cannulated screw fixation and plate fixation for dis-placed intra-articular calcaneus fracture: a meta-analysis of randomized controlled trials. Int J Surg 2016;34:64–72.

Sinus Tarsi Approach with Subcutaneously Delivered Plate Fixation for Displaced Intra-Articular Calcaneal Fractures

Glenn M. Weinraub, DPM[a,b,c,d,*], Marissa S. David, DPM[e]

KEYWORDS

- Calcaneus • Displaced intra-articular calcaneus fracture
- Minimally invasive approach • Sinus tarsi approach • Plate fixation

KEY POINTS

- Operative fixation of Sanders type II, III, and IV displaced intra-articular calcaneal fractures is recommended to achieve the best possible long-term functional outcomes.
- The goal of operative fixation is to restore articular congruency, calcaneal height, width, and alignment.
- The sinus tarsi approach allows for direct reduction of the posterior facet of the subtalar joint while preserving the soft tissue envelope.
- Plate fixation can be used along with the sinus tarsi approach to provide rigid internal fixation.

 Video content accompanies this article at http://www.podiatric.theclinics.com.

INTRODUCTION

Calcaneal fractures are the most commonly seen tarsal bone fractures with both extra-articular and intra-articular fracture patterns observed.[1] Because of the complex nature and high morbidity associated with displaced intra-articular calcaneal fractures (DIACF), open reduction with internal fixation (ORIF) is generally the recommended

Disclosure Statement: No disclosures.
[a] Department of Orthopaedic Surgery, TPMG-GSAA, San Leandro, CA, USA; [b] Midwestern University, Glendale, AZ, USA; [c] Western University, Pomona, CA, USA; [d] American College of Foot and Ankle Surgeons, Chicago, IL, USA; [e] Kaiser Permanente Santa Clara and GSAA, 710 Lawrence Expressway, Department 140, Santa Clara, CA 95051, USA
* Corresponding author. 2500 Merced Street, San Leandro, CA 94577.
E-mail address: Glenn.M.Weinraub@kp.org

Clin Podiatr Med Surg 36 (2019) 225–231
https://doi.org/10.1016/j.cpm.2018.10.005
0891-8422/19/© 2018 Elsevier Inc. All rights reserved.

treatment, because conservative care leads to long-term disability and loss of function.[2-5] The goal of ORIF is to restore congruency of the subtalar joint as well as restore calcaneal height, width, and alignment. ORIF can be performed through many different approaches with the extensile lateral approach (ELA) being the most widely used. This technique is often preferred for its excellent exposure of the calcaneus allowing for direct reduction of the fracture fragments. However, this approach has a high rate of wound complications, including wound edge necrosis and infection. An infection rate of up to 25% is reported in the literature, which can be exacerbated in high-risk patients, such as those with diabetes, peripheral vascular disease, obesity, tobacco use, and drug use.[6-12] In such patients, a more minimally invasive approach should be considered. The goal of the minimally invasive approach is to achieve appropriate reduction of the fracture while preserving the soft tissue envelope and reducing the rate of wound complications postoperatively.[13] Many different techniques have been described, ranging from percutaneous fixation, arthroscopically assisted percutaneous fixation, external fixation, calcaneoplasty, and minimally invasive open techniques. The most common minimally invasive open technique is the sinus tarsi approach because it allows for direct visualization of the posterior facet of the subtalar joint and the calcaneocuboid joint.[14-16] The smaller linear incision also reduces the incidence of wound-healing complications. This article discusses a minimally invasive technique that uses the sinus tarsi approach in combination with internal fixation using a subcutaneous plate.

TECHNIQUE

The operative reduction takes place after an adequate soft tissue holiday to ensure resolution of edema and the return of hindfoot skin wrinkle lines. Anesthesia is either spinal or general technique. Preferred patient positioning is that of complete lateral decubitus; this is especially helpful if one chooses to use an arthroscopic assistive technique during the operation. A well-padded thigh tourniquet is used.

The incision is placed from the tip of the fibula to the superior calcaneal cuboid articulation (**Fig. 1**). The dissection is carried deep, and the peroneal tendons are identified and retracted (**Fig. 2**). Careful subperiosteal dissection is then performed, taking care to stay superficial to the lateral wall fragment. The goal of dissection is to obtain exposure of the fracture fragments and a bony–soft tissue interval for the purpose of

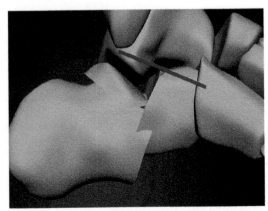

Fig. 1. Incision (*red line*) extends from tip of fibula to the superior calcaneal cuboid articulation.

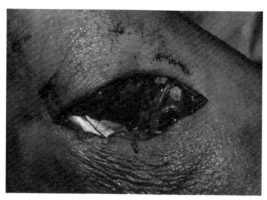

Fig. 2. Initial exposure includes identification of the peroneal tendons and the posterior facet of the subtalar joint.

internal fixation placement. Next, the tuber fragment reduction maneuver is performed. This maneuver ensures both proper heel alignment and decompresses the posterior facet for ease of joint reduction. The authors prefer a modified technique using a 4-mm transcalcaneal tuber pin with a gauze roll bucket handle applied (**Fig. 3**). The bucket handle allows the surgeon to pull the tuber out to length, out of varus, and out of maltranslation with just one hand. The surgeon's other hand (or an assistant) is used to deliver a 2-mm pin from the inferior calcaneal tuber and into the stable sustentaculum fragment, which is oriented from inferior-lateral to superior-medial and left provisionally to maintain tuber alignment. Next, the depressed posterior facet fragment or fragments are rotated back into anatomic alignment and provisionally fixated with small transaxial pins (**Fig. 4**). The posterior facet reduction can also be performed under direct arthroscopic guidance should the surgeon choose (Video 1). Once reduction is deemed appropriate, the primary fragments, including the lateral wall, the posterior facet, and the anterior calcaneal process, are stabilized as one with plate/screw fixation of choice. Once the plate is applied, the posterior facet and calcaneal tuber

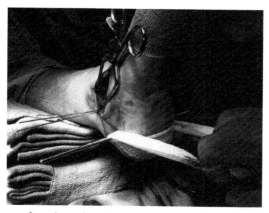

Fig. 3. The authors preferred one-handed technique of calcaneal tuber reduction using a large transaxial pin and a gauze roll bucket handle. The tuber is then provisionally fixated to the sustentaculum tali followed by provisional fixation of the posterior facet with smaller pins.

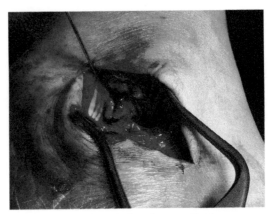

Fig. 4. Completion of reduction and ready for plate application.

can be further stabilized with threaded screws in a nonlag technique (**Fig. 5**). Intraoperative Bröden views are obtained to document good joint reduction (**Fig. 6**). Following closure, the leg is placed into a well-padded posterior splint, and the surgeon's preference of postoperative recovery and therapy is used. The authors prefer 2 weeks of immobilization followed by physiotherapy for a period of 4 to 8 weeks. The patient is kept non-weight-bearing until radiographic evidence of bone healing.

DISCUSSION

Calcaneal fractures are the result of a high-impact axial load on a patient's heel. Consequently, significant disruption of the joint cartilage and calcaneal shape is often seen. Long-term complications of untreated calcaneal fractures can include malunion, posttraumatic subtalar osteoarthritis, chronic foot pain, peroneal tendonitis, and lateral impingement syndrome.[5,17] There has been controversy regarding whether conservative or surgical treatment of DIACF was preferred. Ibrahim and colleagues[17] found that long-term functional and radiographic outcomes at 15 years were similar between patients treated conservatively and operatively. However, Veltmn and colleagues[18] found that patients who underwent ORIF had superior long-term functional outcomes compared with patients who were treated conservatively. This finding is

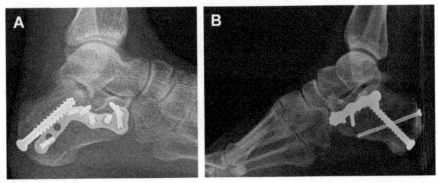

Fig. 5. Two different plate fixation constructs with a Z-shaped plate (*A*) and straight plate (*B*) are demonstrated.

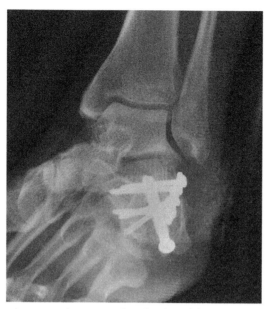

Fig. 6. Bröden view demonstrating anatomic reduction of the posterior subtalar joint facet.

supported by Sanders and colleagues,[19] who used computerized tomography scan to assess fracture reduction radiographically. Patients who had good articular reduction had better clinical results with the exception of type IV fractures, which had poor outcomes even with ORIF. This suggests that surgical treatment gives patients the best chance for a good outcome; however, postoperative complications with the ELA are a major concern. It has been shown that the biggest postoperative complications are infection and poor wound healing. These complications can lead to increased hospital stay, poorer self-reported functional outcomes, and increased incidence of secondary subtalar joint fusion.[6,20,21] Other commonly seen complications with the ELA are injury to the sural nerve or the peroneal tendons. Various minimally invasive approaches have been proposed as a response to these concerns.[13,14,16,20,22] Percutaneous techniques reduce the incidence of these complications; however, the disadvantage is limited exposure of the fracture. Limited exposure leads to difficulty achieving adequate reduction of the fracture and increased use of intraoperative image intensification. There is also an increased incidence of loss of reduction and hardware complication with percutaneous fixation.[23,24] A partially open technique via the sinus tarsi approach provides surgeons with direct visualization of the posterior facet allowing for reduction of the fracture and placement of internal fixation. Another benefit is that it reduces the chance of nervous injury because the incision is made in the internervous plane.[21,25] A meta-analysis of current literature by Yao and colleagues[21] showed that patients who had ORIF through the sinus tarsi approach have a decreased incidence of wound complications compared with the ELA.

COMPLICATIONS/CONCERNS

Abdelazeem and colleagues[14] proposed a minimally invasive technique using the sinus tarsi approach with screw fixation. At 12-month follow-up, no loss of reduction or hardware failure was noted. In addition, 85% of patients were able to return to their preinjury level of work and had improved outcome scores.

Amani and colleagues[15] compared open surgery via ELA to a minimally invasive technique using the sinus tarsi approach. No statistical difference was found between the 2 groups when comparing the postoperative Böhler angle, angle of Gissane, postoperative pain scores, and return to prior activity. The only statistically significant result was the incidence of postoperative wound complications, which was higher in the open surgery group. Jin and colleagues[20] also compared open surgery via ELA to a minimally invasive technique and found a significantly lower incidence of wound complications, decreased postoperative pain, and shorter operative time in the minimally invasive group. At the last follow-up, radiographic data and functional outcome scores were comparable between the 2 groups. This study suggests that you can achieve equally adequate restoration of calcaneal height, width, and length with a minimally invasive approach.

SUMMARY

Although ELA is the gold-standard approach to ORIF of calcaneal fractures, only a small subset of healthy patients are good candidates for this procedure. For those patients who are higher risk for postoperative complications, surgeons should consider a minimally invasive approach like the technique described in this article.

SUPPLEMENTARY DATA

Supplementary data related to this article can be found online at https://doi.org/10.1016/j.cpm.2018.10.005.

REFERENCES

1. Eastwood DM, Gregg PJ, Atkins RM. Intra-articular fractures of the calcaneum: part I: pathological anatomy and classification. J Bone Joint Surg Br 1993;75: 183–8.
2. Griffin D, Parsons N, Shaw E, et al. Operative versus non-operative treatment for closed, displaced, intra-articular fractures of the calcaneus: randomised controlled trial. BMJ 2014;349:g4483. Available at: https://doi.org/10.1136/bmj.g4483. Accessed September 12, 2018.
3. Jiang N, Lin QR, Diao XC, et al. Surgical versus nonsurgical treatment of displaced intra-articular calcaneal fracture: a meta-analysis of current evidence base. Int Orthop 2012;36:1615–22.
4. Sanders R. Displaced intra-articular fractures of the calcaneus. J Bone Joint Surg Am 2000;82:225–50.
5. Sharr PJ, Mangupli MM, Winson IG, et al. Current management options for displaced intra-articular calcaneal fractures: non-operative, ORIF, minimally invasive reduction and fixation or primary ORIF and subtalar arthrodesis. A contemporary review. Foot Ankle Surg 2016;22:1–8.
6. Backes M, Schep NWL, Luitse JSK, et al. The effect of postoperative wound infections on functional outcome following intra-articular calcaneal fractures. Arch Orthop Trauma Surg 2015;135:1045–52.
7. Backes M, Schepers T, Beerekamp S, et al. Wound infections following open reduction and internal fixation of calcaneal fractures with an extended lateral approach. Int Orthop 2014;38:767–73.
8. Benirschke SK, Kramer PA. Wound healing complications in closed and open calcaneal fractures. J Orthop Trauma 2004;18:1–6.

9. Ding L, He Z, Xiao H, et al. Risk factors for postoperative wound complications of calcaneal fractures following plate fixation. Foot Ankle Int 2013;34:1238–44.

10. Koski A, Kuokkanen H, Tukiainen E. Postoperative wound complications after internal fixation of closed calcaneal fracture: a retrospective analysis of 126 consecutive patients with 148 fractures. Scand J Surg 2005;94:243–5.

11. Abidi A, Dhawan S, Gruen GS, et al. Wound healing risk factors after open reduction and internal fixation of calcaneal fractures. Foot Ankle Int 1998;19(12): 856–61.

12. Buch J, Blauensteiner W, Scherafati T, et al. [Conservative treatment of calcaneus fracture versus repositioning and percutaneous bore wire fixation. A comparison of 2 methods]. Unfallchirurg 1989;92(12):595–603.

13. Giannini S, Cadossi M, Mosca M, et al. Minimally-invasive treatment of calcaneal fractures: a review of the literature and our experience. Injury 2016;47:S138–46.

14. Abdelaeem A, Khedr A, Abousayed M, et al. Management of displaced intra-articular calcaneal fractures using the limited open sinus tarsi approach and fixation by screws only technique. Int Orthop 2014;38:601–6.

15. Amani A, Shakeri V, Kamali A. Open surgery vs. minimal invasive methods for calcaneus fractures. Eur J Transl Myol 2018;28:203–9.

16. Arastu M, Sheehan B, Buckley R. Minimally invasive reduction and fixation of displaced calcaneal fractures: surgical technique and radiographic analysis. Int Orthop 2014;38:539–45.

17. Ibrahim T, Rowsell M, Rennie W, et al. Displaced intra- articular calcaneal fractures: 15-year follow-up of a randomized controlled trial of conservative versus operative treatment. Injury 2007;38:848–55.

18. Veltmn ES, Doornberg JN, Stufkens SAS, et al. Long-term outcomes of 1,730 calcaneal fractures: systematic review of the literature. J Foot Ankle Surg 2013; 52:486–90.

19. Sanders R, Fortin P, DiPasquale T, et al. Operative treatment in 120 displaced intra-articular calcaneal fractures. Results using a prognostic computed tomography scan classification. Clin Orthop Relat Res 1993;290:87–95.

20. Jin C, Weng D, Yang W, et al. Minimally invasive percutaneous osteosynthesis versus ORIF for Sanders type II and III calcaneal fractures: a prospective, randomized intervention trial. J Orthop Surg Res 2017;12:10. Available at: https://doi.org/10.1186/s13018-017-0511-5. Accessed September 12, 2018.

21. Yao H, Liang T, Xu Y, et al. Sinus tarsi approach versus extensile lateral approach for displaced intra-articular calcaneal fracture: a meta-analysis of current evidence base. J Orthop Surg Res 2017;12:43. Available at: https://doi.org/10.1186/s13018-017-0545-8. Accessed September 12, 2018.

22. Labbe J, Peres O, Leclair O, et al. Minimally invasive treatment of displaced intra-articular calcaneal fractures using the balloon kyphoplasty technique: preliminary study. Orthop Traumatol Surg Res 2013;99:829–36.

23. Khuran A, Dhillon M, Prabhakar S, et al. Outcome evaluation of minimally invasive surgery versus extensile lateral approach in management of displaced intra-articular calcaneal fractures: a randomised control trial. Foot (Edinb) 2017;31: 23–30.

24. Poigenürst J, Buch J. Treatment of severe fractures of the calcaneus with repositioning and percutaneous wire fixation. Unfallchirurg 1988;91:493–501.

25. Weber M, Lehmann O, Sägesser D, et al. Limited open reduction and internal fixation of displaced intra-articular fractures of the calcaneum. J Bone Joint Surg Br 2008;90:1608–16.

Role of Subtalar Arthroscopy for Displaced Intra-Articular Calcaneal Fractures

Chul Hyun Park, MD, PhD

KEYWORDS

• Calcaneus • Calcaneal fracture • Surgical treatment • Arthroscopy

KEY POINTS

- Subtalar arthroscopy plays an important role in enhancing the reduction of the posterior facet in both percutaneous and open approaches of displaced intra-articular calcaneal fractures.
- In the percutaneous approach, subtalar arthroscopy clearly has a role in surgically managing displaced intra-articular calcaneal fractures; however, this approach is limited to mild-to-moderately displaced fractures.
- In the open approach, including extensile lateral approach and sinus tarsi approach, there is still little evidence of the utility of subtalar arthroscopy alone. Therefore, intraoperative arthroscopy should always be used in conjunction with fluoroscopy to achieve reduction and assess the implant placement.

INTRODUCTION

The treatment of fractures involving the articular surface is always a matter of concern. In particular, the treatment of displaced intra-articular calcaneal fractures (DIACF) is a challenging task for a surgeon because of the irregular anatomy of the calcaneus, complicated coupling with the talus, and delicate soft tissue envelope. Therefore, conservative treatments are generally performed for calcaneal fractures involving the posterior facet.[1–5] On the other hand, the advancements of surgical techniques and equipment have led to a preference for surgery.[6–8]

A well-considered surgical approach is essential for achieving satisfactory outcomes without complications when performing surgery for DIACF. The extensile lateral approach (ELA) has been the most commonly used approach because of its

Funding: This work was supported by the National Research Foundation of Korea (NRF) grant funded by the Korea government (MSIT) (No. 2018R1C1B5036121).
Department of Orthopedic Surgery, Yeungnam University Medical Center, Hyeonchungno 170, Nam-gu, Daegu, 42415, Republic of Korea
E-mail address: chpark77@yu.ac.kr

broad surgical view.[2,9,10] Recently, however, several minimally invasive approaches have been proposed due to the complications associated with ELA, including soft tissue problems, infection, and sural nerve injury. Of the various surgical approaches, the sinus tarsi approach (STA) has gained increasing popularity because of the lower risk of soft tissue complications and sural nerve injury.[11–22] On the other hand, it is difficult to confirm the reduction of the posterior facet using the STA, because the surgical view is quite limited. Even after the ELA, it is also difficult to evaluate the reduction because of the narrow space of the subtalar joint and the irregular shape of the posterior facet.[23]

Subtalar arthroscopy is used widely as a diagnostic and therapeutic tool for intra- or extra-articular pathologic conditions around the subtalar joint.[24,25] Some authors documented the use of subtalar arthroscopy in the surgical treatment of DIACF.[23,26–28] Nevertheless, most articles on the use of subtalar arthroscopy reported arthroscopically assisted percutaneous fixation for extra-articular or less severe intra-articular calcaneal fractures.[23,29–33] Information on the utility of subtalar arthroscopy in the treatment of DIACF is scarce. This article reviews the role of subtalar arthroscopy for DIACF.

ANATOMIC CONSIDERATIONS

An understanding of the irregular anatomic features of the calcaneus and its surrounding structures is essential when deciding the appropriate surgical approach for DIACF. The subtalar joint is a complex articulation from a morphologic and functional point of view.[9] Anatomically, the calcaneus has 4 articulations with its adjacent tarsal bones. Anteriorly, the calcaneus has articulation with the cuboid. Moreover, its surface lies at the distal end of the anterior process of the calcaneus and is biconcave and saddle-shaped.[34] Superiorly, the calcaneus shares 3 articulating surfaces with the talus, including the anterior, middle, and posterior facets. The concave-shaped middle and anterior facets, which are flat, are merged in approximately one-fifth of all cases.[35] The posterior facet is separated from the smaller anterior and middle facets by the calcaneal sulcus, which forms the inferior border of the narrow tarsal canal medially and the wider sinus tarsi laterally.[34] The posterior facet is located in the middle third of the calcaneus. In addition, it is largest of the 3 articulations, the primary load-bearing component of the subtalar joint, and has a complex shape of articulation. The surface is not only convex in the sagittal plane and runs distally and laterally at approximately 45° to the sagittal plane, but it is also concave in the transverse plane.[34] Therefore, the small intra-articular step-off of the posterior facet could be overlooked in Brodén view during surgery.

The talus and calcaneus are held closely together by the strong cervical and interosseous talocalcaneal ligaments.[36] The interosseous ligament, which is found within the tarsal canal, is a stout structure that is shaped like an inverted Y. Its 2 branches (anteromedial and posterolateral) are directed anterolaterally across the sinus tarsi and provide a strong system of intrinsic stabilization to the subtalar joint. Therefore, the space between the talus and calcaneus is narrow, and the posterior facet is difficult to expose when using the STA.

PERCUTANEOUS APPROACH

Less-invasive approaches, including percutaneous, posterior, and sinus tarsi approaches, have been proposed because of the concern regarding wound healing, and they are gaining increasing popularity among surgeons. Less invasive approaches may reduce the risk of postoperative complications and allow for accelerated recovery. The literature supporting the quality of intra-articular reduction achieved by less-invasive approaches is limited, but there are increasing data available.[37]

The percutaneous approach in calcaneal fractures minimizes the incidence of soft tissue-related complications, but carries the risk of inadequate reduction. In the percutaneous approach, reduction of the posterior facet is achieved either by traction, or by percutaneous leverage with an introduced pin. Westhues[29] first described reduction using percutaneous leverage. The procedure gained popularity after the reports by Gissane[30] and Essex-Lopresti,[31] who found it to be particularly useful in tongue-type fractures. Tornetta III[32] expanded the indications for the percutaneous approach to less severe DIACF, such as Sanders type IIC fractures with the posterior facet being displaced as a whole. DeWall and colleagues[33] compared retrospectively the results of a percutaneous approach to an ELA for DIACFs including 125 Sanders types II, III, and IV fractures. They reported improvement of the Bohler angle, loss of reduction at healing, reduction of the calcaneus width, and a similar need for late subtalar fusion in both approaches. In addition, the incidence of deep infection and wound complications was significantly lower in the percutaneous approach.

The challenge of the percutaneous approach is the potential inability to restore the normal anatomy because of the limited exposure of the fracture site. Therefore, arthroscopic assistance can help restore the articular surface. When combining the percutaneous approach with arthroscopic assistance, the indications for the percutaneous approach may be expanded to Sanders type 2A and 2B fractures.[23,38] This combined approach has been called by various names, including percutaneous arthroscopically assisted fixation,[38] percutaneous arthroscopic calcaneal osteosynthesis,[39] arthroscopic-assisted percutaneous screw fixation,[40] arthroscopic reduction and percutaneous fixation,[41] and subtalar arthroscopic-guided percutaneous fixation.[42] In this article, the combined approach is called an arthroscopically assistant percutaneous approach (AAPA). Rammelt and colleagues[43] reviewed 33 patients who underwent the AAPA using the anterolateral and posterolateral portals for Sanders type IIA and IIB calcaneal fractures. They reported satisfactory clinical and radiographic results with no wound complications at the final follow-up, and concluded that the percutaneous approach appears to be preferable over an open reduction and plate fixation in appropriately selected cases of mildly displaced type II fractures. In addition, they highlighted that this approach is unsuitable for uniform application to all types of calcaneal fractures because of the considerable risk of inadequate joint reduction in fractures. The percutaneous approach clearly has a role in the surgical management of DIACF, but this approach must be selected carefully for mild-to-moderately displaced fractures.

SINUS TARSI APPROACH

The STA is the representative less-invasive approach for DIACF. The rationale behind the STA is to reduce any soft tissue dissection while still allowing fracture reduction and stabilization. The STA does not violate the angiosomes of the soft tissue around the lateral wall of the calcaneus. As the STA allows direct visualization of the posterior facet, reduction can be performed with minimal incision through the sinus tarsi, and soft tissue injury can be also reduced. Theoretically, the STA can be used in Sanders type 2 fractures that are not severely comminuted because of the limited surgical view.[22] This approach allows for the fixation of anterior and posterior fragments using screws or a low-profile plate if needed, and decreases the dissection and elevation of the peroneal tendons, thereby theoretically lowering the risk of postoperative tendon problems, such as irritation and subluxation.[44] The risk of postoperative sural nerve injury is also reduced, because the sural nerve is largely avoided during the surgical incision.[44]

In the STA, a 4 cm incision is commonly made over the sinus tarsi along a line from the tip of the fibula to the base of the fourth metatarsal. This incision can be modified to various lengths depending on the fracture characteristics and combined injury. This incision can be extended posteriorly to the visualization and treatment of dislocated peroneal tendons when a peroneal tendon dislocation is accompanied. In addition, the incision can be used later when subtalar arthrodesis is required.[44]

Several studies have reported good clinical and radiographic outcomes and a low incidence of complications for STA,[11–22] despite the varying approach sites, length of incision, and fracture fixation method. Kikuchi and colleagues[15] reviewed 22 calcaneal fractures treated using a limited STA. They used a range of fixation devices including a one-third tubular plate with screws, a combination locking/nonlocking plate with screws, K-wires, or large, fully threaded cannulated screws. In all cases, the Böhler angle and calcaneal width were restored. Three cases (13.6%) of superficial wound infection were managed with local wound care and oral antibiotics, and 1 patient underwent revision surgery for symptomatic hardware removal. Park and colleagues[22] performed a computed tomography (CT)-based study of 20 Sanders type 2 calcaneal fractures treated using an STA and fixation using 4.0 mm cancellous screws and percutaneous 7.0 mm cannulated screws. CT scans were obtained immediately postoperatively and at 12 months after surgery to evaluate the reduction of the posterior facet. Reduction of the posterior facet was graded as good and excellent (ie, step-off <1 mm, defect <5 mm, angulation <5°) in 15 cases (75%) on the immediately postoperative CT, and no loss of reduction was observed by CT obtained 12 months after surgery. A systematic review with 8 case series reporting on 256 patients was conducted to access the results of studies using an STA or modified STA for the treatment of DIACF in 2011.[19] Overall, 75% of patients managed with STA had good-to-excellent outcomes, and wound complications were observed in 4.8% of cases. The investigator concluded that the results of an STA were similar or more favorable than an ELA.

Difficulty in restoring the calcaneal width is the main disadvantage of STA. The ELA can offer the facility of applying an overall compressive force to the lateral calcaneus using a conventional or anatomic plate. On the other hand, performing lateral plating can be a challenge when carrying out the STA because of the limited exposure of the posterior facet.[22] If the calcaneal width is not restored to its normal extent, the distance between the fibular epiphysis and calcaneus narrows and introduces the risk of lateral impingement (Fig. 1). Weber and colleagues[20] reported pain in the subfibular area in 5 (20.8%) out of 24 cases treated using the STA. This was attributed to impingement by screws. In all cases, the pain disappeared after screw removal. Park and Lee[22] compared the calcaneal width of the injured and uninjured side after surgery in 20 DIACFs, and the width of the injured side was significantly greater at the last follow-up. Moreover, 5 cases (25%) developed pain in the subfibular area after weight bearing; the pain disappeared in all cases after removing the screws. They highlighted that symptoms induced by lateral impingement could occur when the STA is chosen and should be taken into consideration.

The detailed surgical procedures of the STA will be described later in this article.

SUBTALAR ARTHROSCOPY

Subtalar arthroscopy was first described by Parisien and Vangsness in 1985.[45] They described their experimental experience of subtalar arthroscopy in 6 cadaver

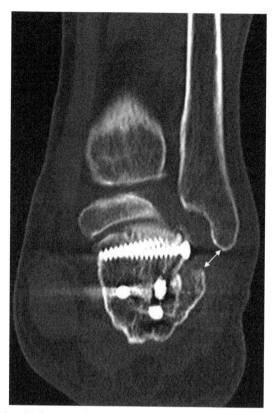

Fig. 1. Postoperative CT showing the reduced distance between the lateral malleolus and calcaneus lateral wall due to an unreduced calcaneal width. Double headed arrow indicates the distance between the lateral malleolus and the protruded calcaneus lateral wall.

specimens and used anterior and posterior portals to approach the posterior facet of the subtalar joint using a 2.7 mm arthroscope. Frey and colleagues[46] introduced the middle portal for subtalar arthroscopy in 1994. They discussed the safety of the anterior, middle and posterior portals by measuring their distance from the neurovascular structures. After its introduction, subtalar arthroscopy has been used as a diagnostic and therapeutic tool for various intra- or extra-articular pathologic conditions.[25] The indications for its application are expanding continuously to include different diagnostic and therapeutic purposes.

In subtalar arthroscopy, the lateral malleolus and Achilles tendon are the anatomic landmarks for portal placement. Three portals, including the anterolateral, centrolateral (or middle), and posterolateral portals, are commonly used (**Fig. 2**).[24] The anterolateral portal is placed 2 cm anterior and 1 cm distal to the tip of the lateral malleolus. The centrolateral portal is placed just anterior to the tip of the lateral malleolus. The posterolateral portal is placed at the tip of the lateral malleolus or 0.5 cm proximal, which is close to the Achilles tendon, to avoid injury to the sural nerve.

Small instruments are needed to visualize the posterior facet because of the tightness of the subtalar joint. A 2.7 mm 30° arthroscope is commonly used for subtalar arthroscopy. A 70° arthroscope can be useful for looking around corners and facilitating instrumentation. A 1.9 mm 30° arthroscope is recommended in subtalar joints that are too tight to allow a 2.7 mm arthroscope.

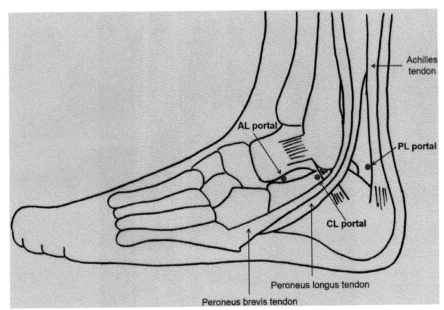

Fig. 2. Illustration showing the placements of anterolateral (AL), centrolateral (CL), and posterolateral (PL) portals.

ROLE OF SUBTALAR ARTHROSCOPY

Arthroscopy has been used for several years in the foot and ankle to diagnose and treat pathologic conditions. Its role has also evolved over time and continues to expand. Compared with open surgery, subtalar arthroscopy has some advantages in the treatment of DIACF.[42] First, the damaged posterior facet can be observed in real time and visualized up close. Second, small bony fragments, cartilage, and hematoma lodged in the medial portion of the subtalar joint can be removed with a shaver. Third, joint penetration of screws can be detected easily. Fourth, intraoperative Brodén views have been used to visualize the posterior facet that cannot be observed directly. On the other hand, Brodén views using fluoroscopy provide inaccurate information owing to the low resolution and complex shape of the subtalar joint[23]; therefore, a small intra-articular step-off can be overlooked by fluoroscopy. Arthroscopy not only allows simpler detection of the intra-articular step-off, but also makes it easier to identify angulation of the posterior facet after the reduction, which is difficult to detect in intraoperative Brodén views (**Fig. 3**).

The use of arthroscopy in the treatment of DIACFs was first performed in open reductions and internal fixation through an ELA.[23,26] In 2002, Gavlik and colleagues[26] first described the use of open subtalar arthroscopy in an open reduction and internal fixation through an ELA for DIACFs. They reported that despite the seemingly exact reduction, minor step-off (between 1 and 2 mm) was detected arthroscopically in 12 cases (25.5%). In the same year, the same authors introduced the AAPA in DIACFs.[38] They concluded that AAPA offers a precise assessment of the articular surface and allows anatomic reduction while adhering to the principles of minimally invasive surgery. Since then, several authors have reported good clinical and radiographic outcomes with a low complication rate for AAPA using a range of portals and different sized arthroscopes (**Table 1**).[23,39–43]

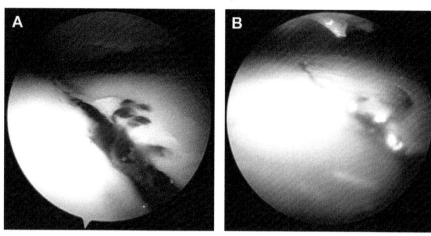

Fig. 3. Arthroscopic image showing angulation of the posterior facet after reduction (*A*). Arthroscopic image showing a good reduction of the posterior facet without angulation after reattempting the reduction (*B*).

Few reports can be found on the arthroscopic-assisted open reduction and internal fixation in the treatment of DIACF (**Table 2**).[27,28] Recently, Park and Yoon[27] reported the utility of open subtalar arthroscopy in surgical treatment using an STA for DIACF. They evaluated the fracture reduction using intraoperative fluoroscopy in the first 23 fractures and in the latter 23 fractures using intraoperative fluoroscopy and subtalar arthroscopy. They reported that the combined approach using fluoroscopy and subtalar arthroscopy showed better reduction of the posterior facet on CT than using fluoroscopy alone, even though no significant differences in the short-term clinical results and complication rate were observed.

Consensus is lacking regarding which fracture configuration is best treated with arthroscopy alone, fluoroscopy alone, or with the combined approach using fluoroscopy and arthroscopy. Arthroscopy allows excellent visualization of the articular surface, but fluoroscopy has better roles in an evaluation of the calcaneal width and height, determination of the screw length, and restoration of the calcaneocuboid joint congruity. Therefore, intraoperative arthroscopy should always be used in conjunction with fluoroscopy to achieve reduction and assess implant placement.

Some problems related to the subtalar arthroscopy procedures used in the treatment of calcaneus fractures can be encountered.[27] First, it is difficult to insert the arthroscope into the subtalar joint without iatrogenic chondral injury because of the narrow space of the subtalar joint. Generally, a small-diameter (2.4 mm or 2.7 mm) arthroscope is used to overcome this problem. In addition, the exertion of varus stress via the Steinmann pin used for reduction of the tuberosity fragment can facilitate the approach. Some authors highlighted the horizontal insertion of the arthroscope to the subtalar joint for easier insertion and good visualization of the posterior facet.[27] Therefore, an additional portal in front of the operative incision is required in some cases. Second, there are concerns regarding the use of arthroscopy, including the potential for increased setup and surgery time, a steep learning curve, and increased initial costs. On the other hand, Rammelt and colleagues[23] reported that open arthroscopy is less time-consuming than a complete intraoperative Brodén series with plain radiographs. Park and Yoon[27] also showed that the operative time was similar in treatment with fluoroscopy alone and with combined fluoroscopy and arthroscopy. Third, there

Table 1
Studies with arthroscopically assistant percutaneous approach

Author, Year	Study Design	Sander's Type	Patients (n)	Mean Follow-up (mo)	Using Arthroscope	Using Portals	Δ of Bohler Angle (°)	AOFAS Score	STJ Fusion	Complications
Gavlik et al,[26,38] 2002	Retrospective	II	10	<24	1.9 mm, 0° or 4.0 mm, 30°	AL, PL	11.2	93.7	NR	1 (HR)
Rammelt et al,[23] 2002	Retrospective	II	18	15	1.9 mm, 0°	AL, PL	12.7	92.1	0	1 (HR)
Rammelt et al,[43] 2010	Retrospective	II	24	29	2.7 mm, 30°	AL, CL, PL	13	92.1	0	2 (HR)
Woon et al,[42] 2011	Prospective	II	22	33	2.4 mm, 0°	AL, CL	17.1	84.2	0	1 (HR), 1 (WI)
Sivakumar et al,[41] 2014	Retrospective	II, III, IV	13	14.3	2.9 mm, 30°	AL, CL	18.3	87.8	0	1 (HR)
Pastides et al,[39] 2015	Prospective	II, III	33	24	4.0-mm, 30°	AL, CL, PL	12.3	72.2	0	2 (HR), 1 (WI)
Yeap et al,[40] 2016	Retrospective	II, III	15	16.9	2.7-mm, 30°	AL, CL, PL	15.9	86.7	0	1 (HR)

Abbreviations: AL, anterolateral; AOFAS, American Orthopaedic Foot and Ankle Society; CL, centrolateral; HR, hardware removal; NR, not recorded; PL, posterolateral; STJ, subtalar joint; WI, wound infection.
Data from Refs.[23,38–43]

Table 2
Studies with arthroscopically assistant open reduction and internal fixation

Author, Year	Study Design	Sander's Type	Patients (n)	Mean Follow-up (mo)	Using Approach	Using Arthroscope	Δ of Bohler Angle (°)	AOFAS Score	STJ Fusion	Complications
Gavlik et al,[26,38] 2002	Retrospective	II, III, IV	47	NR	ELA	1.9-mm, 0° or 4.7-mm, 30°	NR	NR	NR	NR
Rammelt et al,[23] 2002	Retrospective	II, III, IV	59	NR	ELA	1.9-mm, 0° or 4.0-mm, 30°	NR	NR	NR	NR
Schuberth et al,[28] 2009	Retrospective	I, II, III	24	56.1	STA	4.0-mm, 70°	10.5	NR	NR	NR
Park et al,[27] 2018	Retrospective	II	23	15.9	STA	2.4-mm, 30°	14.7	91.7	0	2 (HR), 3 (TNI)

Abbreviations: AOFAS, American Orthopaedic Foot and Ankle Society; ELA, extensile lateral approach; STA, sinus tarsi approach; HR, hardware removal; NR, not recorded; STJ, subtalar joint; TNI, transient nerve injury.
Data from Refs.[23,26–28]

is a risk of complications related to arthroscopy, such as neurologic injury, tendon injury, compartment syndrome due to fluid extravasation, and pulmonary embolism.[47] Although the risk of these complications is rare, they can be devastating and should be noted.

AUTHOR'S PREFERRED TECHNIQUE

The authors commonly use an arthroscopy-assisted STA for joint depression-type fractures of Sanders type 2A and 2B with moderate-to-severe depression of the posterior facet. AAPA is preferred in tongue-type fractures and joint depression-type fractures with mild depression. Here, the arthroscopy-assisted STA for DIACF is described.

The patient is placed in the lateral decubitus position using a beanbag, and a tourniquet is applied at the thigh. Fluoroscopy is brought in from the end of the bed, and the fluoroscopy equipment and arthroscopic equipment are placed dorsal and oblique to the patient (**Fig. 4**).

A 4.5 mm Steinmann pin or a 5-mm Schanz pin is inserted into the calcaneal tuberosity before making a skin incision. Gentle distraction with varus and valgus levering is applied manually to reduce the length of the calcaneus and overcome the shortening of the soft tissues. A 4 cm incision is made along the tarsal sinus from the tip of the lateral malleolus to the calcaneocuboid joint along the tarsal sinus (**Fig. 5**). If accompanied by a dislocation of the peroneal tendons, the incision is extended posteriorly along the lateral malleolus to confirm and repair the superior peroneal retinaculum (**Fig. 6**). Careful dissection is performed between the peroneal tendons and the sinus fat pad, preserving the sural nerve. The extensor digitorum brevis is retracted proximally, and the peroneal tendons are retracted plantarly. To expose the fracture site, the lateral capsule is incised, and the calcaneal fibular ligament is mobilized and retracted posteriorly; the floor of the sinus tarsi is then debrided. To expose the posterior portion of the posterior facet widely, the calcaneal fibular ligament can be detached on the tip of the lateral malleolus and repaired using a suture anchor after fracture fixation (**Fig. 7**). After removing the hematoma and small bone fragments, the impacted posterolateral fragment is elevated using a small curette or freer and reduced using the inferior surface of the talus as a template. After reduction of the posterolateral fragment, 2 Kirschner wires are inserted through the

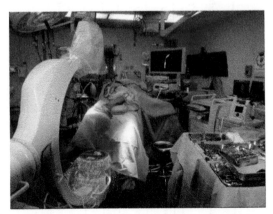

Fig. 4. Positioning of the surgical bed, fluoroscopy, fluoroscopy, and arthroscopy equipment.

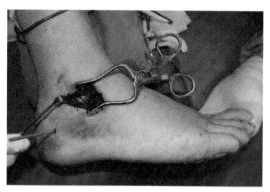

Fig. 5. Conventional sinus tarsi approach.

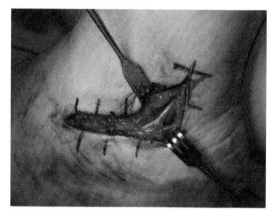

Fig. 6. Extended sinus tarsi approach for a peroneal tendons dislocation combined with a calcaneal fracture.

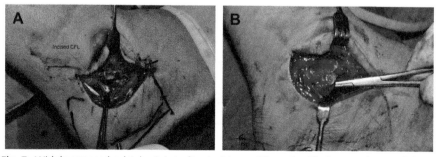

Fig. 7. Widely exposed subtalar joint after incising a CFL at the fibular attachment (*A*). Repaired CFL using a 2.7 mm suture anchor (*B*).

fragment directed toward the sustentaculum to provisionally hold the reduced fragment. Reduction of the posterior facet is first evaluated using Brodén view by fluoroscopy (**Fig. 8**). After this step, reduction of the posterior facet is confirmed again using open subtalar arthroscopy through the previous skin incision or additional anterolateral portal (**Fig. 9**). To decrease the thickness of the arthroscope, an arthroscopic cannula is generally not used, and dry arthroscopy is performed. A small-diameter (2.4 mm) arthroscope is introduced by applying varus stress using the Steinmann pin that is used for reduction of the tuberosity fragment. The reduction is confirmed by advancing the arthroscope from the front to the back of the posterior facet. In particular, the posterior part of the posterior facet, which is difficult to confirm with Brodén view, is checked thoroughly. If the residual step-off is confirmed arthroscopically, a fine correction is carried out under direct arthroscopy guidance (**Fig. 10**). After obtaining satisfactory reduction of the posterior facet, definite fixation is performed using 2 2.7 mm cortical screws with the lag technique (**Fig. 11**). Valgus and downward stresses are then applied using a Steinmann pin or a Schanz pin to correct any hindfoot alignment and restore the calcaneal height. If varus alignment of the hindfoot or collapsed calcaneal height is not reduced, a small elevator or lamina spreader is placed under the posterior facet fragment through the fracture line and manipulated to ascertain the amount of reductions necessary (**Fig. 12**). The calcaneal width is restored by laterally compressing the heel, which is an important step in preventing lateral impingement (**Fig. 13**). Lateral compression of the heel should not be performed unless the articular fragments are reduced completely, because this would make further reduction of the articular fragments difficult. Once good reduction is achieved, 2 or 3 7 mm cannulated fully threaded screws are inserted from the posterior heel to the anterior process for fixation between the anterior process and posterior facet fragments (**Fig. 14**). Reduction, hindfoot alignment, and screw positions are checked using fluoroscopy, and wound closure is performed with interrupted sutures.

A short leg splint is applied for 4 weeks postoperatively. Passive and active motion exercises of the ankle and subtalar joint are initiated the day after surgery. Weight

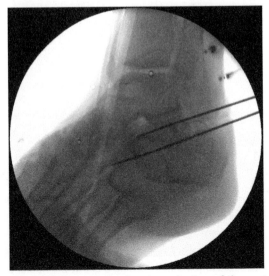

Fig. 8. Intraoperative Brodén view confirming the reduction of the posterior facet.

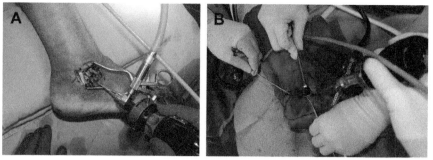

Fig. 9. Confirming the reduction of the posterior facet using open subtalar arthroscopy through the previous skin incision (*A*) or additional anterolateral portal (*B*).

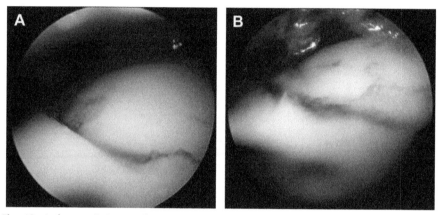

Fig. 10. Arthroscopic image showing a step-off of more than 1 mm (*A*). After additional reduction, achieving an anatomic reduction without step-off (*B*).

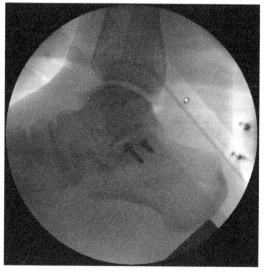

Fig. 11. Definite fixation of the posterior facet fragments using 2 2.7-mm cortical screws with the lag technique.

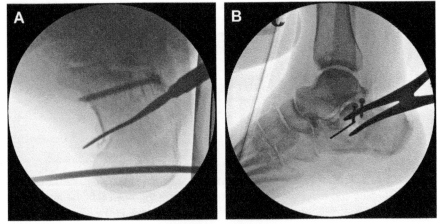

Fig. 12. Reduction of residual hindfoot varus using a freer (*A*). Reduction of a collapsed calcaneal height using a lamina spreader placed under the posterior facet fragment through the fracture site (*B*).

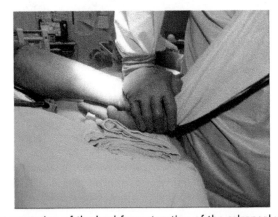

Fig. 13. Lateral compression of the heel for restoration of the calcaneal width.

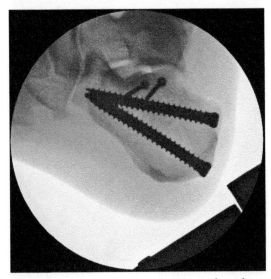

Fig. 14. Fixation between the anterior process and posterior facet fragments using 2 7 mm cannulated fully threaded screws.

bearing is commenced at 6 to 8 weeks after surgery depending on the bone quality and type of fracture.

SUMMARY

This article highlighted the important role of subtalar arthroscopy in enhancing the reduction of the posterior facet in both percutaneous and open approaches of DIACF. In the percutaneous approach, arthroscopy clearly has a role in surgically managing DIACF; however, AAPA must be selected carefully for mild-to-moderately displaced fractures. In the open approach, including ELA and STA, there is still little evidence of the utility of subtalar arthroscopy. Therefore, intraoperative arthroscopy should always be used in conjunction with fluoroscopy to achieve reduction and assess the implant placement.

REFERENCES

1. Sanders R. Intra-articular fractures of the calcaneus: present state of the art. J Orthop Trauma 1992;6(2):252–65.
2. Sanders R, Fortin P, DiPasquale T, et al. Operative treatment in 120 displaced intraarticular calcaneal fractures. Results using a prognostic computed tomography scan classification. Clin Orthop Relat Res 1993;(290):87–95.
3. McLaughlin HL. Treatment of late complications after os calcis fractures. Clin Orthop Relat Res 1963;30:111–5.
4. Lindsay WR, Dewar FP. Fractures of the os calcis. Am J Surg 1958;95(4):555–76.
5. Rowe CR, Sakellarides HT, Freeman PA, et al. Fractures of the os calcis: a long-term follow-up study of 146 patients. JAMA 1963;184(12):920–3.
6. Kocis J, Stoklas J, Kalandra S, et al. Intra-articular calcaneal fractures. Acta Chir Orthop Traumatol Cech 2006;73(3):164–8.
7. Kundel K, Funk E, Brutscher M, et al. Calcaneal fractures: operative versus nonoperative treatment. J Trauma 1996;41(5):839–45.
8. Sanders R. Displaced intra-articular fractures of the calcaneus. J Bone Joint Surg Am 2000;82(2):225–50.
9. Benirschke SK, Sangeorzan BJ. Extensive intraarticular fractures of the foot. Surgical management of calcaneal fractures. Clin Orthop Relat Res 1993;292: 128–34.
10. Buckley R, Tough S, McCormack R, et al. Operative compared with non-operative treatment of displaced intra-articular calcaneal fractures: a prospective, randomized, controlled multicenter trial. J Bone Joint Surg Am 2002; 84-A(10):1733–44.
11. Ebraheim NA, Elgafy H, Sabry FF, et al. Sinus tarsi approach with trans-articular fixation for displaced intra-articular fractures of the calcaneus. Foot Ankle Int 2000;21(2):105–13.
12. Femino JE, Vaseenon T, Levin DA, et al. Modification of the sinus tarsi approach for open reduction and plate fixation of intra-articular calcaneus fractures: the limits of proximal extension based upon the vascular anatomy of the lateral calcaneal artery. Iowa Orthop J 2010;30:161–7.
13. Geel CW, Flemister AS Jr. Standardized treatment of intra-articular calcaneal fractures using an oblique lateral incision and no bone graft. J Trauma 2001;50(6): 1083–9.
14. Hospodar P, Guzman C, Johnson P, et al. Treatment of displaced calcaneus fractures using a minimally invasive sinus tarsi approach. Orthopedics 2008;31(11): 1112–7.

15. Kikuchi C, Charlton TP, Thordarson DB. Limited sinus tarsi approach for intra-articular calcaneus fractures. Foot Ankle Int 2013;34(12):1689–94.
16. Kline AJ, Anderson RB, Davis WH, et al. Minimally invasive technique versus an extensile lateral approach for intra-articular calcaneal fractures. Foot Ankle Int 2013;34(6):773–80.
17. Mostafa MF, El-Adl G, Hassanin EY, et al. Surgical treatment of displaced intra-articular calcaneal fracture using a single small lateral approach. Strategies Trauma Limb Reconstr 2010;5(2):87–95.
18. Nosewicz T, Knupp M, Barg A, et al. Mini-open sinus tarsi approach with percutaneous screw fixation of displaced calcaneal fractures: a prospective computed tomography-based study. Foot Ankle Int 2012;33(11):925–33.
19. Schepers T. The sinus tarsi approach in displaced intra-articular calcaneal fractures: a systematic review. Int Orthop 2011;35(5):697–703.
20. Weber M, Lehmann O, Sagesser D, et al. Limited open reduction and internal fixation of displaced intra-articular fractures of the calcaneum. J Bone Joint Surg Br 2008;90(12):1608–16.
21. Gupta A, Ghalambor N, Nihal A, et al. The modified Palmer lateral approach for calcaneal fractures: wound healing and postoperative computed tomographic evaluation of fracture reduction. Foot Ankle Int 2003;24(10):744–53.
22. Park CH, Lee DY. Surgical treatment of sanders type 2 calcaneal fractures using a sinus tarsi approach. Indian J Orthop 2017;51(4):461–7.
23. Rammelt S, Gavlik JM, Barthel S, et al. The value of subtalar arthroscopy in the management of intra-articular calcaneus fractures. Foot Ankle Int 2002;23(10):906–16.
24. Park CH, Kim SY, Kim JR, et al. Arthroscopic excision of a symptomatic os trigonum in a lateral decubitus position. Foot Ankle Int 2013;34(7):990–4.
25. Munoz G, Eckholt S. Subtalar arthroscopy: indications, technique and results. Foot Ankle Clin 2015;20(1):93–108.
26. Gavlik JM, Rammelt S, Zwipp H. The use of subtalar arthroscopy in open reduction and internal fixation of intra-articular calcaneal fractures. Injury 2002;33(1):63–71.
27. Park CH, Yoon DH. Role of subtalar arthroscopy in operative treatment of sanders type 2 calcaneal fractures using a sinus tarsi approach. Foot Ankle Int 2018;39(4):443–9.
28. Schuberth JM, Cobb MD, Talarico RH. Minimally invasive arthroscopic-assisted reduction with percutaneous fixation in the management of intra-articular calcaneal fractures: a review of 24 cases. J Foot Ankle Surg 2009;48(3):315–22.
29. Westhues H. Eine neue Behandlungsmethode der Calcaneusfrakturen. Zugleich ein Vorschlag zur Behandlung der Talusfrakturen. Zentralbl Chir 1935;35:995–1002.
30. Gissane W. News notes: proceedings of the British Orthopedic Association. J Bone Joint Surg Am 1947;29:254–5.
31. Essex-Lopresti P. The mechanism, reduction technique, and results in fractures of the os calcis. Br J Surg 1952;39(157):395–419.
32. Tornetta P 3rd. The Essex-Lopresti reduction for calcaneal fractures revisited. J Orthop Trauma 1998;12(7):469–73.
33. DeWall M, Henderson CE, McKinley TO, et al. Percutaneous reduction and fixation of displaced intra-articular calcaneus fractures. J Orthop Trauma 2010;24(8):466–72.
34. Hall RL, Shereff MJ. Anatomy of the calcaneus. Clin Orthop Relat Res 1993;290:27–35.

35. Keener BJ, Sizensky JA. The anatomy of the calcaneus and surrounding structures. Foot Ankle Clin 2005;10(3):413–24.
36. Pisani G, Pisani PC, Parino E. Sinus tarsi syndrome and subtalar joint instability. Clin Podiatr Med Surg 2005;22(1):63–77, vii.
37. Sharr PJ, Mangupli MM, Winson IG, et al. Current management options for displaced intra-articular calcaneal fractures: nonoperative, ORIF, minimally invasive reduction and fixation or primary ORIF and subtalar arthrodesis. A contemporary review. Foot Ankle Surg 2016;22(1):1–8.
38. Gavlik JM, Rammelt S, Zwipp H. Percutaneous, arthroscopically-assisted osteosynthesis of calcaneus fractures. Arch Orthop Trauma Surg 2002;122(8):424–8.
39. Pastides PS, Milnes L, Rosenfeld PF. Percutaneous arthroscopic calcaneal osteosynthesis: a minimally invasive technique for displaced intra-articular calcaneal fractures. J Foot Ankle Surg 2015;54(5):798–804.
40. Yeap EJ, Rao J, Pan CH, et al. Is arthroscopic assisted percutaneous screw fixation as good as open reduction and internal fixation for the treatment of displaced intra-articular calcaneal fractures? Foot Ankle Surg 2016;22(3):164–9.
41. Sivakumar BS, Wong P, Dick CG, et al. Arthroscopic reduction and percutaneous fixation of selected calcaneus fractures: surgical technique and early results. J Orthop Trauma 2014;28(10):569–76.
42. Woon CY, Chong KW, Yeo W, et al. Subtalar arthroscopy and fluorosocopy in percutaneous fixation of intra-articular calcaneal fractures: the best of both worlds. J Trauma 2011;71(4):917–25.
43. Rammelt S, Amlang M, Barthel S, et al. Percutaneous treatment of less severe intraarticular calcaneal fractures. Clin Orthop Relat Res 2010;468(4):983–90.
44. Hsu AR, Anderson RB, Cohen BE. Advances in surgical management of intra-articular calcaneus fractures. J Am Acad Orthop Surg 2015;23(7):399–407.
45. Parisien JS, Vangsness T. Arthroscopy of the subtalar joint: an experimental approach. Arthroscopy 1985;1(1):53–7.
46. Frey C, Gasser S, Feder K. Arthroscopy of the subtalar joint. Foot Ankle Int 1994; 15(8):424–8.
47. Gonzalez TA, Macaulay AA, Ehrlichman LK, et al. Arthroscopically assisted versus standard open reduction and internal fixation techniques for the acute ankle fracture. Foot Ankle Int 2016;37(5):554–62.

Joint-Sparing Surgical Management of Sanders IV Displaced Intra-Articular Calcaneal Fractures

Thomas S. Roukis, DPM, PhD

KEYWORDS

- Arthrodesis • CALCANAIL • Fusion • Open reduction • Sanders classification
- Surgery • Subtalar joint • Trauma

KEY POINTS

- Displaced intra-articular calcaneal fractures of the Sanders IV fracture pattern are life-altering events with historically poor clinical and functional outcomes.
- Controversy persists between open reduction with internal fixation, primary subtalar arthrodesis, and open reduction with internal fixation alone for Sanders IV fracture pattern.
- Incision healing complications are exceedingly common with either reconstruction when performed through a lateral extensile incision, which has prompted the development of minimally invasive techniques to reduce the known incision healing problems.
- The CALCANAIL allows operative intervention to be performed with a shorter delay between injury and surgery.
- Subtalar arthrodesis can be performed, either at the time of the index surgery if the joint is nonreconstructable, or in delayed manner if post-traumatic arthritis develops.

INTRODUCTION

The severe, permanent, life-altering consequences of sustaining a displaced intra-articular calcaneal fracture (DIACF) have been recognized since antiquity.[1] In 1935, Conn[2] stated that DIACFs were "...a serious and disabling injury in which the end results are incredibly bad." In 1942, Bankart[3] stated, "The results of treatment of crush fractures of the [calcaneus] are rotten ...It would seem that the best result that can be expected from a fracture of the [calcaneus] involving the [subtalar] joint is a completely stiff but painless foot of a good shape, and with free movement of the ankle joint." The difficulty in obtaining any semblance of normal calcaneal morphology through

Disclosure: Consultant for DePuy Synthes, FH ORTHO, Integra and Novastep. Royalties received from CrossRoads Extremity, Novastep and Stryker Orthopaedics.
Orthopaedic Center, Gundersen Health System, 1900 South Avenue, La Crosse, WI 54601, USA
E-mail address: tsroukis@gundersenhealth.org

operative intervention was highlighted in 1963 when McLaughlin[4] stated that fixation of DIACF was as effective as "...nailing a custard pie to the wall." More recently Rammelt and colleagues[5] stated that, "The poorest treatment results are reported after open surgical treatment that failed to achieve anatomic reconstruction of the calcaneum and its joints, thus combining the disadvantages of operative and nonoperative treatment. The crucial question, therefore, is not only whether to operate or not but also when and how to operate on calcaneal fractures if surgery is decided" (**Fig. 1**). Anderson[6] asked if DIACF remained the "unsolved" or was the "unsolvable" intra-articular orthopedic injury. Although the answer to this question remains a matter for conjecture, what is clear is that, despite carefully planned and executed operative intervention by trauma/foot and ankle surgeons experienced with treating DIACF, few clinical, radiographic, and intra-operative findings reliably predict which patient will develop chondrolysis and post-traumatic degenerative subtalar joint disease or what anatomic structure(s) is/are responsible for chronic postoperative pain (**Fig. 2**).[7–13]

The severity of comminution based on computerized tomography (CT) imaging, specifically the Sanders IV type fractures,[14] which, by definition, have at least 3 fracture lines across the posterior subtalar facet, have historically resulted in persistent pain, poor functional outcomes, and high need for secondary subtalar

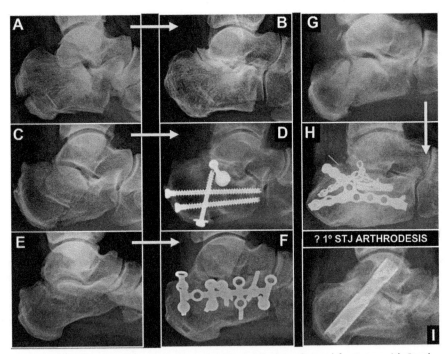

Fig. 1. Lateral heel radiographs of displaced intra-articular calcaneal fractures with Sanders IV fracture patterns treated nonoperatively (*A, B*), with closed manipulation and cannulated screw fixation (*C, D*), open reduction with internal fixation through and extensile lateral incision using a perimeter (*E, F*), and Y-shaped plate (*G, H*), all demonstrating loss of reduction back to the original index deformity. Lateral heel radiograph following closed manipulation and primary subtalar arthrodesis using a rigid, intramedullary locked nail demonstrating maintained calcaneal morphology (*I*). Note: arrows indicate corresponding pre- and post-fracture care images.

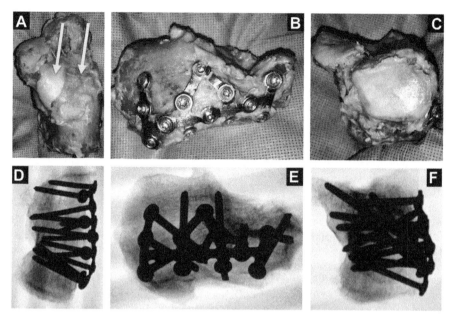

Fig. 2. Postmortem dissection of the right calcaneus following remote open reduction with internal fixation using a perimeter plate and screw construct through a lateral extensile incision. Photographs of the calcaneus demonstrating extensive chondrolysis and avascular changes to the subchondral bone of the lateral aspect of the posterior subtalar joint (*yellow arrow*) compared with the preserved sustentaculum fragment (*blue arrow*) (*A*). Lateral (*B*) and anterior-posterior (*C*) photographs, as well as axial (*D*), lateral (*E*), and anterior-posterior (*F*) radiographs of the calcaneus demonstrating malunion with varus angulation, loss of height, and incongruency of the posterior subtalar joint.

joint arthrodesis with nonoperative and operative intervention.[15–19] Primary arthrodesis of the subtalar joint without fracture reduction for treatment of DIACF was originally proposed by Van Stockum in 1912,[20] followed by Stulz in 1930,[21] who recommended open reduction and primary subtalar joint arthrodesis. The benefit of an open reduction with internal fixation (ORIF) and primary subtalar joint arthrodesis in this severe injury pattern is based on several factors. First, a large prospective Canadian study demonstrated that Sanders IV DIACF cases have a 5.5 times higher likelihood of requiring subtalar arthrodesis compared with fractures of lesser complexity, specifically a Sanders II type pattern.[22] Second, Sanders IV DIACF cases account for between one-half and two-thirds of the late subtalar arthrodeses performed in large cohort groups with DIACF.[14,22,23] Third, 25% of the Sanders IV DIACF cases require arthrodesis within 2 years of surgery.[22] Fourth, the functional outcomes and pain reduction of those undergoing delayed subtalar arthrodesis after ORIF are generally high,[14,24,25] especially when the initial treatment was operative with good restoration of the calcaneal morphology.[26] Finally, the overall financial burden and patient disability associated with are surgeries are lessened with a single operative intervention and associated convalescence.[27] All told, and at face value, ORIF and primary subtalar arthrodesis appear to be the treatment of choice for Sanders IV DIACF with nonreconstructable articular surfaces. However, a systematic review of publications between 1990 and 2010 demonstrated that Sanders IV DIACF cases are, in fact, rare, and the percentage of all patients undergoing operative fixation with a primary subtalar arthrodesis averaged only 5%.[28]

Infante and colleagues[29] described performing ORIF and primary subtalar joint arthrodesis in 33 (6%) of 503 DIACF cases between 1991 and 1997 at their level 1 trauma center. All injuries were caused by high-energy etiologies and included 10 open fractures and 16 with fractures additional ipsilateral foot or ankle injuries. The mean patient age was 40 years. The decision to perform arthrodesis was determined preoperatively in 17 patients based on radiographic injury pattern and in 13 patients intraoperatively based on nonreconstructable posterior subtalar joint pattern. Twenty-eight (85%) of the subtalar arthrodeses required bone graft augmentation, with 21 autogenous iliac crest bone graft and 7 allografts. Fracture fixation was performed with plate(s) and screws, and the subtalar arthrodesis was performed with 6.5 and/or 8 mm screws. Three (9.1%) patients were lost to follow-up. The mean follow-up was 38 months. Two patients developed nonunion, with the remaining developing osseous union 4 month postoperatively. Complications developed in 10 patients, including 7 wounds, of which 4 developed osteomyelitis requiring debridement and intravenous antibiotics, with 2 of these ultimately requiring below-knee amputation. Since this initial publication a limited, several additional case series have been reported. Jung and colleagues[30] performed 10 ORIF and primary subtalar arthrodeses in 9 patients for Sanders IV DIACF due to inability to reconstruct the subtalar joint. The follow-up period was 20.3 month months. At final follow-up, the mean visual analog pain scale was 3.9 on a 10-point scale; 50% of the patients were satisfied, and 80% were able to return to their previous employment at a mean of 8.4 months. Morales and colleagues[31] performed 6 ORIF and primary subtalar arthrodeses with autogenous bone graft and a single cannulated 7 mm screw for nonreconstructable DIACF between 1997 and 2002. The follow-up period was 20.3 months. Similar to the previous reports, wound complications occurred in 50% of patients; osseous union occurred in all patients at a mean of 4 months, and they all returned to work within 6 month postoperatively. Holm and colleagues[32] performed 17 ORIF and primary subtalar arthrodeses using a variety of fixation constructs for nonreconstructable DIACF. The follow-up period was 34 months, at which time the mean visual analog pain scale was 1.9 on a 10-point scale. There were no nonunions. They determined a significant improvement in patient-reported functional outcomes with restoration of the Böhler and lateral talo-calcaneal angles.

More recent literature supports the use of closed manipulation, percutaneous external fixation distractor-assisted ligamentotaxis/tendinotaxis to restore calcaneal morphology, intra-osseous indirect subtalar joint surface reduction, subtalar joint arthrodesis, and stabilization with a rigid, locked intra-medullary nail contained within the calcaneus and talus.[33-39] Representative implants that incorporate these features include the CALCANAIL (FH Orthopedics, Chicago, Illinois) and VIRA Calcaneal System (Biomet Spain Orthopedics, SL, Valencia, Spain). Of these, the CALCANAIL is the only implant available in the United States for clinical use. Simon and colleagues[33] conducted a prospective, nonrandomized clinical study of 69 displaced intra-articular calcaneal fractures treated with the CALCANAIL. Out of a cohort of 19 Sanders IV fracture patterns, a primary subtalar arthrodesis was performed with the CALCANAIL fusion nail in 6 patients, and an additional 2 patients underwent a delayed secondary subtalar joint arthrodesis within the first year after surgery. The patients returned to work within 6 months. The American Orthopedic Foot and Ankle Surgery Hindfoot-Ankle Scoring Scale (AOFAS-HFAS) was 75.6/92-points, which was similar to the 78/92-points identified by Holm and colleagues[32] The ability to also convert to a secondary subtalar joint arthrodesis using dedicated nail extraction reamers and the larger-diameter 12 mm CALCANAIL makes this an attractive salvage option because of the minimal soft-tissue dissection, ability to distract and compress the subtalar joint as indicated, pack bone graft into the hollow central chamber, and deliver a robust intramedullary locked nail. Using the VIRA system for closed reduction and primary subtalar joint arthrodesis, López-Oliva and colleagues[36–38] have published on a series of patient cohorts. López-Oliva and colleagues[37] performed primary subtalar joint fusions for 53 DIACFs with Sanders IIIAB and IV fracture patterns. At 12 month after surgery, the mean AOFAS-HFAS score was 76.6 points. Patients rated their outcomes as very good (26%), good (62%), and fair-poor (12%). López-Oliva and colleagues[36] prospectively evaluated 37 DIACFs with Sanders IIIAB and IV fracture patterns treated with primary subtalar joint fusions using the VIRA system. At 12 months after surgery, the mean AOFAS-HFAS score was 75.43 points. Patients rated their outcomes as very good/good (84%) and fair/poor (16%). Subtalar joint arthrodesis was achieved in all cases, and only 1 case required bone grafting. There were 7 (23%) cases of hindfoot valgus malalignment demonstrated but no other complications documented. In the largest study to date, López-Oliva and colleagues[38] prospectively evaluated 169 DIACFs with Sanders IIIAB and IV fracture patterns treated with primary subtalar joint fusions using the VIRA system in a purely patient with active workers compensation claims. At the end of follow-up, the mean AOFAS-HFAS score was 77.26 points. Patients rated their outcomes as excellent (25%), good (64%), mild 7%, and poor (4%). Subtalar joint arthrodesis was achieved in all cases, and only 3 cases required bone grafting. Major complications occurred in 5 patients, and deep infection occurred in 1 patient. Similar to the CALANAIL, López-Oliva and colleagues[39] described successful secondary subtalar joint arthrodesis using the VIRA system in 11 cases. Complications consisted of 2 subtalar nonunions requiring reoperation and impaction bone grafting to achieve union. Only 3 patients were unable to return to their prior occupation, with the remainder returning to work at 4.1 months after surgery. At the end of follow-up, the mean AOFAS-HFAS score was 71.6 points.

Because patient outcome following operative treatment of DIACF is directly correlated with surgeon experience,[7] and ORIF with primary subtalar arthrodesis is so rarely performed[28] but involves a variety of surgical approaches and fixation methods,[29–36] how can a surgeon be expected to maintain a highly complex and perishable skill set particular to the Sanders IV fracture pattern?[7,40] In reality, treatment options should ideally be tailored to the fracture's unique personality, the surgeon's most consistently reliable operative intervention, and the individual patient-specific requirements.[8,10]

JOINT-SPARING SURGICAL MANAGEMENT OF SANDERS IV DISPLACED INTRA-ARTICULAR CALCANEAL FRACTURES

Chen and colleagues[41] described performing ORIF through a lateral extensile incision in 26 Sanders III and 32 Sanders IV fracture pattern DIACFs. Mean time from injury to surgery was 10 days (range: 7–14 days). The mean patient age was 29.5 years (range: 17–58 years). The mean follow-up was 13 months (range: 6–24 months). Complications developed in 8 patients, including 2 incisions with superficial necrosis, 2 instances of advanced subtalar joint post-traumatic arthrosis, and 4 feet with chronic pain. According to the Maryland Foot Score, the results were excellent in 23 patients, good in 27 patients, fair in 5 patients, and poor in 3 patients. They concluded that ORIF through the lateral extensile approach was an effective method for operative management of Sanders III and IV fracture patterns. Buckley and colleagues[24] conducted a prospective, randomized, multicenter trial at 4 level 1 trauma centers in Canada to compare long-term outcomes between ORIF and ORIF with primary subtalar joint arthrodesis for treatment of Sanders IV fracture patterns. The study involved 26 fractures treated between 2004 and 2011 and followed for a minimum of 2 years and maximum of 7 years. The ORIF group had a lateral extensile exposure and the posterior facet fragments were secured with compression screws and/or threaded Kirschner wires followed by nonlocking plate fixation of the lateral wall. The ORIF with primary subtalar joint arthrodesis was performed in the same manner for calcaneal fracture fixation, and then the posterior facet of the subtalar joint was resected followed by autogenous iliac crest bone graft or femoral head allograft bone graft when large osseous defects were encountered. Fixation of the subtalar joint arthrodesis was with large partially and/or fully threaded 7.3 mm compression screws. There was no demonstrable statistically significant difference between the patient-related outcome measures performed between the 2 groups; however, both groups scored poorly on general health outcomes. This reflects the severity of this Sanders IV DIACF injuries and the detrimental impact these injuries have on a patient's life. Only 1 patient of the 17 ORIF procedures performed underwent a secondary subtalar joint arthrodesis. The only noticeable difference was that the ORIF group average nonweightbearing period was 10 weeks compared with the ORIF with primary subtalar joint arthrodesis, which was 6 weeks. Similarly, Woo and colleagues[42] conducted a prospective, randomized study to compare long-term outcomes between ORIF and ORIF with primary subtalar joint arthrodesis for treatment of Sanders IV fracture patterns. The study involved 22 fractures treated between 2003 and 2013 and followed for a minimum of 18 months (mean of 34.6 months). There was no demonstrable statistically significant difference between the patient-related outcome measures performed between the 2 groups; however, patient satisfaction was higher in the ORIF group with primary subtalar joint arthrodesis. Secondary subtalar arthrodesis was performed for 5 patients in the ORIF group within 2 years. Although ORIF can achieve restoration of calcaneal morphology and posterior subtalar joint articular cartilage shape, what is the cost for using the lateral extensile incision and volume of internal fixation required to achieve stable fixation (**Fig. 3**)? Closed manipulation, intraosseous reduction, and rigid intramedullary locked nail fixation using the CALCANAIL have been developed to address these concerns.

Simon and colleagues[33] conducted a prospective, nonrandomized clinical study of 69 displaced intra-articular calcaneal fractures treated with the CALCANAIL. Out of a cohort of 19 Sanders IV fracture patterns, an intraosseous reduction and CALCANAIL fixation were performed in 13 patients, with only 2 patients ultimately undergoing a delayed secondary subtalar joint arthrodesis within the first year after surgery. The American Orthopedic Foot and Ankle Surgery Hindfoot-Ankle Scoring Scale (AOFAS-HFAS) was 80/92 points. Falis and Pyszel[34] evaluated 18 Sanders IV fracture patterns treated with an intraosseous reduction, and CALCANAIL fixation was performed in 7 patients. Similarly, Weiss and colleagues[43] evaluated 19 Sanders IV fracture patterns threated with an intraosseous reduction and CALCANAIL fixation. Neither of these studies had a patient treated with later subtalar arthrodesis and concluded that CALCANAIL was a safe and reliable implant for use in Sanders IV fracture patterns. Fascione and colleagues[44] evaluated 2 Sanders IV fracture patterns treated with an intraosseous reduction and CALCANAIL fixation, with 1 of the patients with poor reduction of the calcaneal morphology and posterior subtalar joint facet requiring delayed subtalar arthrodesis at 11 months after surgery. It should be noted that this patient was the author's second case performed in his series of 15 DIACFs, and the poor outcome was most likely because of this severe fracture pattern being treated early in the

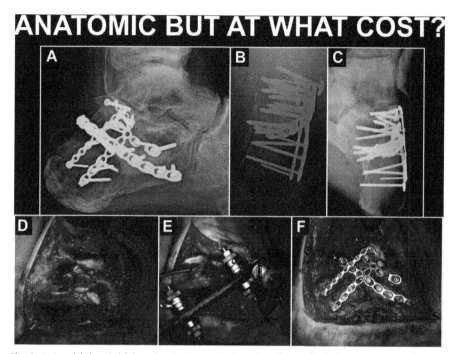

Fig. 3. Lateral (*A*), axial (*B*) and anterior-posterior (*C*) radiographs following open reduction and internal fixation through an extensile lateral incision (*D*) and temporary external fixation assisted calcaneal realignment (*E*) and stabilization with multiple plates and screws (*F*) for a Sanders IV fracture pattern. Although the articular surfaces have been restored anatomically and the calcaneal morphology recreated the extensive soft-tissue dissection and volume of internal fixation required begs the question, "anatomic but at what cost?" since secondary surgery can with be fraught with potential complications.

author's learning curve with the CALCANAIL rather than the CALCANAIL system itself.

SURGICAL TECHNIQUE: OPEN REDUCTION WITH INTERNAL FIXATION

Surgery must be delayed until the soft tissues are conditioned for surgery, and this delay can approach 2 weeks when extensive hemorrhagic blistering is present (**Fig. 4**). One should perform this procedure with the patient in the lateral or lateral-decubitus position. Tourniquet control is usually necessary. An extensive L-shaped incision is employed as described by Borrelli Jr and Lashgari,[45] respecting the arterial supply to the full-thickness soft-tissue flap,[46,47] which is elevated subperiosteally as a full-thickness flap being careful to avoid iatrogenic injury to the Sural nerve and its branches.[48,49] It is useful to employ a tube-to-bar external fixation device as an intraoperative reduction tool through placement of a half-pin in the talar neck and the second in the calcaneal tuber. Manual distraction of the calcaneus with an open compressor-type clamp allows for restoration of the calcaneal length, height, and rotation.[50–52] The smaller articular fragments are provisionally fixated with a smooth Kirschner wire and then secured with a minifragment small diameter screw(s) (**Fig. 5A–C**). Although controversial for use in Sanders II and III DIACFs, cancellous bone allograft is frequently employed to fill the osseous void and support the posterior

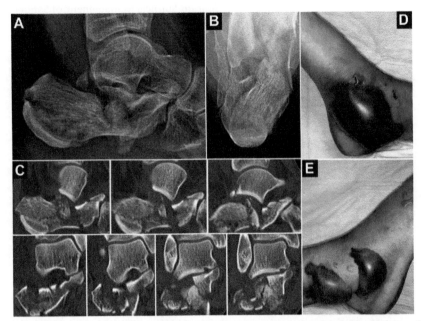

Fig. 4. Lateral (*A*) and axial (*B*) heel radiographs and computed tomography (CT) imaging (*C*) demonstrating a Sanders IV fracture pattern. Clinical photographs of the medial (*D*) and lateral (*E*) soft tissues 2 days after the index injury demonstrating extensive hemorrhagic fracture blistering.

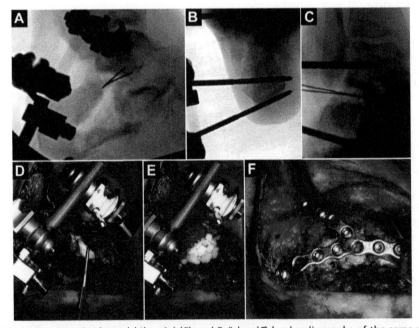

Fig. 5. Intraoperative lateral (*A*), axial (*B*) and Bröden (*C*) heel radiographs of the same patient shown in **Fig. 4** demonstrating restoration of the calcaneal morphology with use of a temporary external fixation device as an intraoperative reduction tool. Intraoperative photographs demonstrating re-insertion of the comminuted osteo-articular fragments (*D*), filling of the osseous void within the neutral triangle with cancellous bone allograft (*E*), and stabilization with a Y-shaped calcaneal plate and screw construct (*F*).

facet osteoarticular fragments (**Fig. 5**D, E).[53] A calcaneal specific Y-shaped (**Fig. 5**F)[54] or perimeter plate[14] is then applied to the lateral calcaneal wall and secured with, ideally, bicortical nonlocking screws; however, on occasion it is necessary to employ locking screws to provide enhanced stability.[55] A closed suction drain is placed, and the surgical incision is closed in 1 layer, with attention paid to minimize tension at the apex of the full-thickness flap, thereby limiting wound-healing complications.[56] Because of the frequency of wound healing complications at the apex of the incision, Wang and colleagues[57] described the use of a proximally based abductor digiti minimi muscle flap that they proposed would enhance vascularity to this delicate region and provide soft-tissue coverage over the plate and screw fixation. Should a wound develop over the apex of the incision, the use of a pie-crusting skin meshing technique,[58] coupled with hardware removal, can reliable provide durable soft-tissue coverage (**Fig. 6**).

SURGICAL TECHNIQUE: CLOSED MANIPULATION, INTRAOSSEOUS REDUCTION AND CALCANAIL FIXATION

One should perform this procedure with the patient placed in the prone position under general anesthesia. Tourniquet control is not necessary. Under intraoperative C-arm image intensification, a guide wire with stopper is driven into the posterior tuberosity

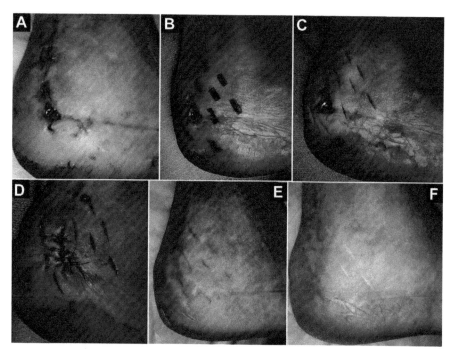

Fig. 6. Clinical photographs of the lateral heel of the same patient shown in **Figs. 4** and **5** demonstrating exposed plate and screw hardware at the apex of the extensile lateral incision (*A*). Intraoperative photographs of the lateral heel demonstrating planned pie-crusting skin meshing incisions (*B*) that are developed full-thickness (*C*) and allow for expansion of the soft tissues so the wound can be closed primarily (*D*). Clinical photographs of the lateral heel at 6 weeks (*E*) and 2 years (*F*) after surgery demonstrating excellent soft tissue coverage and minimal scar formation.

aiming toward the lateral process of the talus, since the critical angle of Gissane is unrecognizable with Sanders IV fracture patterns (**Fig. 7**A), and on the axial view within the center of the calcaneal tuberosity axis and parallel to any varus deformity present (**Fig. 7**B). A 3.2 mm Kirschner wire is then placed bicortical through the positioning square perpendicular to the to the guide wire. A second 3.2 mm Kirschner wire is then placed bicortically into and perpendicular to the talar neck. The caspar-type distraction device is then placed over the Kirschner wires in the calcaneus and talus and secured with small thumbscrews. Once secured to the Kirschner wires, the large thumbscrew on the caspar-type device is dialed to distract apart the calcaneal fracture fragments and open the subtalar joint until the calcaneal tuber has been brought out of varus, as well as the length and height restored (**Fig. 7**C, D). Next, the hollow trephine is placed over the guide wire with a stopper and advanced under image intensification to just beneath the subchondral bone of the posterior facet (**Fig. 7**E). If subchondral bone of the posterior facet is unrecognizable, as is often the case, then the trephine should be advanced into the region of the neutral triangle within the body of the calcaneus only to minimize further disruption or inadvertent fragmentation of the periarticular fragments. The trephine is removed and the cylindrical bone graft contained within it saved for later use; however, the bone graft may be of limited volume because of the degree of osseous fragmentation occurring with Sanders IV fracture

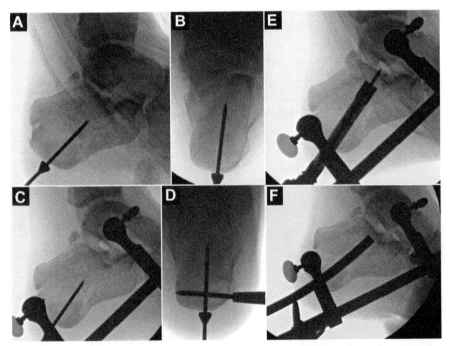

Fig. 7. Intraoperative lateral (*A*) and axial (*B*) image intensification views demonstrating guide wire with stopper followed by caspar-type distractor-assisted restoration of the calcaneal morphology including the length and height on the lateral (*C*) view, as well as width and frontal plane angulation on the axial (*D*) view. Intraoperative lateral view demonstrating insertion of the hollow reamer to the level of subchondral bone (*E*). Intraoperative lateral view demonstrating intraosseous reduction of the articular segments of the posterior subtalar joint with a curved tamp (*F*).

patterns. Next, the largest of the posterior facet fragments are sequentially reduced using the inferior surfaces of the talus as a template with a combination of curved, spatula-shaped and straight tamps placed through the working chamber created by the trephine (**Fig. 7**F). Smaller fragments are freed from their impaction within the calcaneal body, but only if doing so does not cause further damage to the larger fragments that should take priority. Although dependent on the fracture pattern, most commonly the medial constant fragment is first elevated followed by the lateral and then central fragments with C-arm image intensification employed to track the reduction until the subtalar joint line is congruent. The length of the 10 mm diameter fracture nail is measured with available lengths being 45, 50, and 55 mm, and, once selected, the oblong window is packed with the previously harvested autogenous bone graft from the trephine, or, if necessary, an allograft (ConformFlex, Synthes USA Products, LLC, West Chester, Pennsylvania) can be employed. The nail is then introduced through the working chamber (**Fig. 8**A) and locked with 2 bicortical cannulated, threaded locking screws placed through the alignment targeting device. It is critical to have these screws obtain sound purchase within the sustentaculum tali fragment and the posterior calcaneal tuber, which have the densest cortical bone available and provide the soundest stabilization (**Fig. 8**B, C). A plantarly oriented aiming arm allows for placement of an optional oblique screw through the oblong window of the CALCANAIL to increase rotational stability and secure larger posterior calcaneal tuber

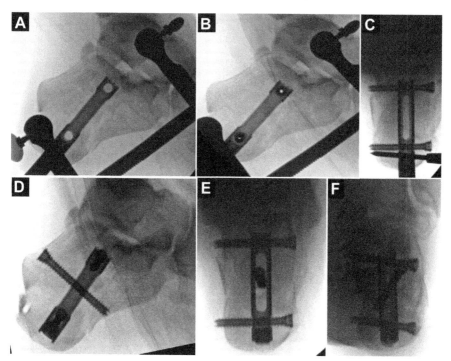

Fig. 8. Intraoperative lateral view demonstrating insertion of the CALCANAIL to a depth just deep to the posterior subtalar joint facet subchondral bone (*A*). Intraoperative lateral (*B*) and axial (*C*) views following placement of the lateral-to-medial oriented locking screws. Intraoperative lateral (*D*), axial (*E*) and Bröden (*F*) image intensification views following final CALCANAIL insertion demonstrating maintenance of calcaneal morphology and near anatomic reduction of the posterior subtalar joint facet.

fracture fragments (**Fig. 8D–F**). Additional independent screws can be placed free-hand through the largest fragments to provide additional stability. If the osseous void is significant within the calcaneal body, it can be backfilled with an injectable fiber-reinforced calcium phosphate bone void filler (Norian Drillable Inject, DePuy Synthes USA Products, LLC, West Chester, Pennsylvania) to fill the bone defect after the calcaneus has been stabilized with the CALCANAIL (**Fig. 9**). Once the interlocking screws are placed, an end-cap is inserted to facilitate removal if necessary, and then the distractor is removed. The patient is placed in a well-padded sterile dressing from toes to knee, with the addition of a posterior splint to maintain the foot in slight plantarflexion to minimize pull of the Achilles tendon. Patients who are reliable remain in a dressing until skin incision has healed, which routinely occurs at the 2-week visit, followed by placement into a nonarticulated immobilization boot, with range of motion initiated. Nonweightbearing is maintained for 6 weeks followed by gradual return to full weightbearing and transition to shoe gear with serial surveillance radiographs obtained to assess osseous healing (**Fig. 10**).

COMPLICATIONS AND CONCERNS

The most common, and feared, complications associated with ORIF of Sanders IV pattern DIACF are wound-related skin flap necrosis, dehiscence, and secondary

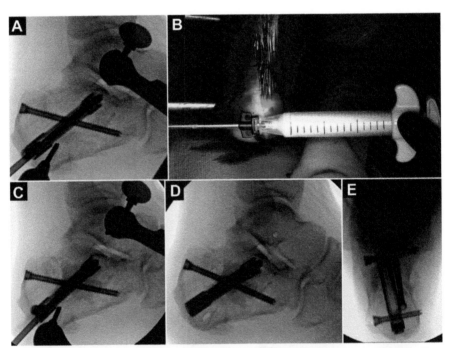

Fig. 9. Intraoperative lateral radiograph (*A*) and photograph (*B*) of an injectable fiber-reinforced calcium phosphate bone void filler demonstrating backfilling of the osseous void within the neutral triangle of the calcaneus (*C*). Intraoperative lateral (*D*) and axial (*E*) views demonstrating complete filling of the osseous void with the fiber-reinforced calcium phosphate. This particular patient was floridly noncompliant and began immediately ambulating distances upon hospital discharge; still, the fracture reduction was maintained, and complete osseous healing occurred.

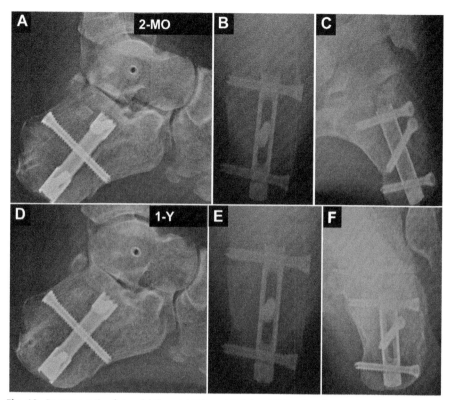

Fig. 10. Postoperative lateral (*A*), axial (*B*) and Bröden (*C*) heel radiographs of the same patient shown in **Figs. 7** and **8** at 6 weeks after surgery demonstrating maintained calcaneal morphology and posterior subtalar joint reduction with osteo-cartilaginous segment of bone retained within the calcaneal body. Postoperative lateral (*D*), axial (*E*), and Bröden (*F*) heel radiographs at 1 year after surgery demonstrating narrowing and sclerosis of the posterior subtalar joint but unchanged calcaneal morphology and posterior subtalar joint reduction with incorporation of the free osteo-cartilaginous segment of bone. This heavy laborer returned to full-time employment at 3 months after surgery and had mild, activity-related pain, swelling, and stiffness at his 1-year follow-up treated with minimal conservative efforts.

deep infection, as these sequelae can result in below-knee amputation.[48,56] Failure to restore calcaneal morphology, especially malunion, results in poor clinical outcomes and complicates future surgery.[5] Inadequate restoration of the posterior subtalar joint facet articular surface and avascular necrosis of the posterior subtalar joint facet with associated chondrolysis are unfortunately common and most often prompt the need for a delayed subtalar joint arthrodesis.[13,15,17] Although closed manipulation, intraosseous reduction, and CALCANAIL fixation offer several advantages over plate and screw fixation, a learning curve exists and is dependent on the surgeon's familiarity with the techniques employed, including use of external distraction devices, percutaneous maneuvers performed with heavy reliance on intraoperative image intensification, and operating with the patient in the prone position. Available publications using the CALCNAIL for ORIF and ORIF with primary subtalar arthrodesis are sparse, and most studies have some patients with unacceptable joint reduction that required secondary arthrodesis.[33–35,44]

SUMMARY

Sanders IV DIACFs represent the most challenging fracture pattern for the most challenging fracture in the foot. The damage sustained to the soft tissues, bone, and cartilage are irreversible and life-altering. ORIF with primary subtalar arthrodesis represents the last definitive operative procedure. Unfortunately, the available literature for this approach using the extensile lateral approach demonstrates only fair clinical outcomes; moderate degrees of pain, swelling, and stiffness; and, in general, the ability to return to employment between 6 and 12 months after surgery. Similar outcomes occur with ORIF for Sanders IV fracture patterns using an extensile lateral incision. The complications associated with the extensile lateral incision are obviated with the use of minimally invasive reduction techniques that preserve the soft tissues, and stout internal fixation provided by the CALCANAIL device is capable of allowing early operative intervention even with compromised soft tissues and bilateral Sanders IV DIACF (**Figs. 11** and **12**). The existing studies specific to Sanders IV fracture patterns, including use of the CALCANAIL fusion nail for ORIF with primary subtalar arthrodesis and the CALCANIL fracture nail for ORIF, offer promising results and the unique ability to convert to arthrodesis if the posterior facet is determined to be nonreconstructable interoperatively, as well as, no documented wound healing problems or infectious complications. However, with surgical expenses under greater scrutiny, more literature is needed to better study the cost-benefit analysis of this device compared with contemporary fixation options when performing ORIF for Sanders IV fracture

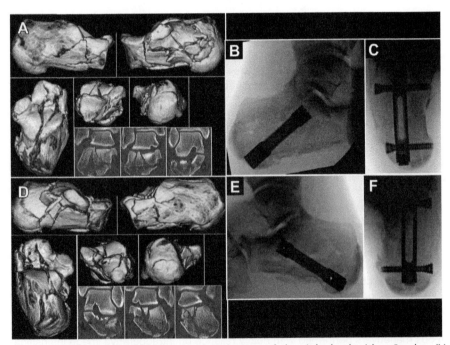

Fig. 11. Three-dimensional and coronal CT images of the right heel with a Sanders IV fracture pattern sustained bilateral and image intensification views following final CALCANAIL insertion demonstrating maintenance of calcaneal morphology and near anatomic reduction of the posterior subtalar joint facet for the right (*A–C*) and left (*D–F*) heels.

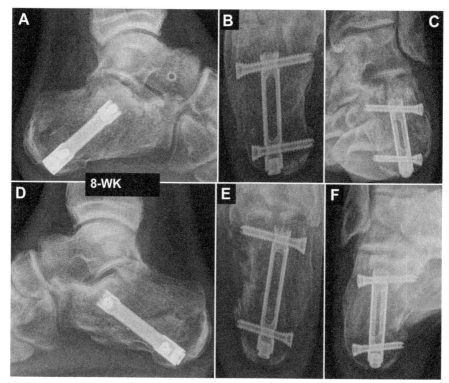

Fig. 12. Weightbearing postoperative lateral, axial, and Bröden heel radiographs demonstrating maintained calcaneal morphology and posterior subtalar joint reduction for the right (*A–C*) and left (*D–F*) heels. This particular homeless, illicit drug-dependent patient left the hospital against medical advice and resurfaced 8 weeks later, at which time lateral, axial, and Bröden heel radiographs confirmed that fracture reduction was unchanged; the posterior subtalar joint alignment was maintained, and progressive osseous healing occurred.

patterns, as well as comparing this approach to ORIF with primary subtalar joint arthrodesis using the CALCANAIL fusion nail.

REFERENCES

1. Wells C. Fractures of the heel bones in early and prehistoric times. Practitioner 1976;217:294–8.
2. Conn H. The treatment of fractures of the os calcis. J Bone Joint Surg 1935;17: 392–405.
3. Bankart A. Fractures of the os calcis. Lancet 1942;240:175.
4. McLaughlin H. Treatment of late complications after os calcis fractures. Clin Orthop Relat Res 1963;30:111–5.
5. Rammelt S, Sangeorzan B, Swords M. Calcaneal fractures: should we or should we not operate? Indian J Orthop 2018;52:220–30.
6. Anderson R. The unsolvable fracture? Tech Foot Ankle Surg 2014;3:205.
7. Guerado E, Bertrand ML, Cano JR. Management of calcaneal fractures: what have we learnt over the years? Injury 2012;43:1640–50.

8. Sharr P, Mangupli MM, Winson IG, et al. Current management options for displaced intra-articular calcaneal fractures: non-operative, ORIF, minimally invasive reduction and fixation or primary ORIF and subtalar joint arthrodesis: a contemporary review. Foot Ankle Surg 2016;22:1–8.

9. Eckstein C, Kottmann T, Füchmeier B, et al. Long-term results of surgically treated calcaneal fractures: an analysis with a minimum follow-up period of twenty-years. Int Orthop 2016;40:365–70.

10. Koutserimpas C, Magarakis G, Kastanis G. Complications of intra-articular calcaneal fractures in adults: key points for diagnosis, prevention and treatment. Foot Ankle Spec 2016;9:534–42.

11. Gotha HE, Zide JR. Current controversies in management of calcaneal fractures. Orthop Clin North Am 2017;48:91–103.

12. Sanders R. Current concepts review: displaced intra-articular fractures of the calcaneus. J Bone Joint Surg Am 2000;82:225–50.

13. Ball S, Jadin K, Allen R, et al. Chondrocyte viability after intra-articular calcaneal fractures in humans. Foot Ankle Int 2007;28:665–8.

14. Sanders R, Fortin P, DiPasquale T, et al. Operative treatment in 120 displaced intraarticular calcaneal fractures. Results using a prognostic computed tomography scan classification. Clin Orthop Relat Res 1993;290:87–95.

15. Rammelt S, Zwipp H, Schneiders W, et al. Severity of injury predicts subsequent function in surgically treated displaced intra-articular calcaneal fractures. Clin Orthop Relat Res 2013;471:2885–98.

16. Alexandridis G, Gunning AC, Leenen LP. Patient-reported health-related quality of life after a displaced intra-articular calcaneal fracture: a systematic review. World J Emerg Surg 2015;10:62.

17. Ågren P-H, Mukka S, Tullberg T, et al. Factors affecting long-term treatment results of displaced intraarticular calcaneal fractures: a post hoc analysis of a prospective, randomized, controlled multicenter trial. J Orthop Trauma 2014;28:564–8.

18. D'Almeida V, Devasia T, Kamath A. Functional assessment following open fixation of calcaneal fractures. J Evolution Med Dental Sci 2014;3:10482–9.

19. Griffin D, Parsons N, Shaw E, et al. Operative versus non-operative treatment for closed, displaced, intra-articular fractures of the calcaneus: randomized controlled trial. BMJ 2014;349:g4483.

20. Von Stockum A. Operative Behandlung der Calcaneus-und Talusfraktur. Zentralbl Chir 1912;39:1438–9.

21. Simon R, Stulz E. Operative treatment of compression fractures of the calcaneus. Ann Surg 1930;91:731–8.

22. Csizy M, Buckley R, Tough S, et al. Displaced intraarticular calcaneal fractures: variables predicting late subtalar fusion. J Orthop Trauma 2003;17:106–12.

23. Thermann H, Huefner T, Schratt E, et al. Long-term results of subtalar fusions after operative versus non-operative treatment of os calcis fractures. Foot Ankle Int 1999;20:408–16.

24. Buckley R, Leighton R, Sanders D, et al. Open reduction and internal fixation compared with ORIF and primary subtalar arthrodesis for treatment of Sanders type IV calcaneal fractures: a randomized multicenter trial. J Orthop Trauma 2014;28:577–83.

25. Buckley R, Tough S, McComack R, et al. Operative compared with nonoperative treatment of displaced intra-articular calcaneal fractures. J Bone Joint Surg Am 2002;84:1733–44.

26. Radnay C, Claire M, Sanders R. Subtalar fusion after displaced intra-articular calcaneal fractures: does initial operative treatment matter? J Bone Joint Surg Am 2009;91:541–6.

27. Buckley R. Letter to the editor response: open reduction and internal fixation compared with ORIF and primary subtalar arthrodesis for treatment of Sanders type IV calcaneal fractures: a randomized multicenter trial. J Orthop Trauma 2014;28:e301–3.

28. Schepers T. The primary arthrodesis for severely comminuted intra-articular fractures of the calcaneus: a systematic review. Foot Ankle Surg 2012;18:84–8.

29. Infante A, Heier K, Lewis B, et al. Open reduction internal fixation and immediate subtalar fusion for comminuted intra-articular calcaneal fractures: a review of 33 cases. J Orthop Trauma 2000;14:142–3.

30. Jung H, Kim Y, Jeon S. Primary subtalar arthrodesis for the treatment of intra-articular calcaneal comminuted fractures. J Korean Fract Soc 2006;19:418–23.

31. Morales F, Malvarez J, Belluschi G, et al. Primary subtalar arthrodesis in workers with calcaneal fractures. Rev Ortop Traumatol 2006;50:372–7.

32. Holm J, Laxson S, Schuberth J. Primary subtalar joint arthrodesis for comminuted fractures of the calcaneus. J Foot Ankle Surg 2015;54:61–5.

33. Simon P, Goldzak M, Eschler A, et al. Reduction and internal fixation of displaced intra-articular calcaneal fractures with a locking nail: a prospective study of sixty-nine cases. Int Orthop 2015;39:2061–7.

34. Falis M, Pyszel K. Treatment of displaced intra-articular calcaneal fractures by intramedullary nail: preliminary report. Ortop Traumatol Rehab 2016;18:141–7.

35. Fernandez B, Padiolleau G, Viejo-Fuerte D. Percutaneous osteosynthesis of calcaneus fractures by locked nail Calcanail: functional and anatomical results- a review of 54 cases. Méd Chir Pied 2018;34:1–6.

36. López-Oliva F, Forriol F, Sánchez-Lorente T, et al. Treatment of severe fractures of the calcaneus by reconstruction arthrodesis using the Vira® system: prospective study of the first 37 cases with over 1 year follow-up. Injury 2010;41:804–9.

37. López-Oliva F, Sánchez-Lorente T, Hernández G, et al. Management of comminuted calcaneal fractures by reconstruction-arthrodesis with the Vira system: a prospective study of the first 50 cases with over one-year follow-up. Trauma 2008;19:28–36.

38. López-Oliva F, Sánchez-Lorente T, Fuentes-Sanz A, et al. Primary fusion in worker's compensation intraarticular calcaneus fracture: prospective study of 169 consecutive cases. Injury 2012;43:S73–8.

39. López-Oliva F, Forriol F, Sánchez-Lorente T, et al. Secondary arthrodesis using the Vira system for treating the sequelae of calcaneus fractures. Rev Esp Cir Ortop Traumatol 2010;54:44–9.

40. Kwon J, Diwan A, Susarla S, et al. Effect of surgeon training, fracture, and patient variables on calcaneal fracture management. Foot Ankle Int 2011;32:262–71.

41. Chen Z-W, Yang L-Z, Wu W-T, et al. Treatment of Sanders type III and IV calcaneal fractures with open reduction and internal fixation. Zhongguo Gu Shang 2011;24: 641–4 [in Chinese].

42. Woo SH, Chung H-J, Bae S-Y, et al. Comparative study of open reduction and internal fixation and primary subtalar arthrodesis for Sanders type IV intra-articular calcaneal fractures. J Korean Orthop Assoc 2017;52:49–58.

43. Weiss M, Dolata T, Weiss W, et al. Treatment of intraarticular displaced fractures of the calcaneus bone using nail locked CALCANAIL. J Ed Health Sport 2018;8: 338–45.

44. Fascione F, Di Mauro M, Guelfi M, et al. Surgical treatment of displaced intraarticular calcaneal fractures by a minimally invasive technique using a locking nail: a preliminary study. Foot Ankle Surg 2018. Available at: https://doi.org/10.1016/j.fas.2018.08.004. Accessed August 28, 2018.

45. Borrelli J Jr, Lashgari C. Vascularity of the lateral calcaneal flap: a cadaveric injection study. J Orthop Trauma 1999;13:73–7.

46. Carow J, Carow J, Gueorguiev B, et al. Soft tissue micro-circulation in the healthy hindfoot: a cross-sectional study with focus on lateral surgical approaches to the calcaneus. Int Orthop 2018. https://doi.org/10.1007/s00264-018-4031-7.

47. Donders JCE, Klinger CE, Shaffer AD, et al. Quantitative and qualitative assessment of the relative arterial contributions to the calcaneus. Foot Ankle Int 2018;39:604–12.

48. Li S. Wound and sural nerve complications of the sinus tarsi approach for calcaneal fractures. Foot Ankle Int 2018. https://doi.org/10.1177/1071100718774808.

49. Smyth N, Zachwieja E, Buller L, et al. Surgical approaches to the calcaneus and the sural nerve: there is no safe zone. Foot Ankle Surg 2017. Available at: https://doi.org/10.1016/j.fas.2017.06.005. Accessed August 28, 2018.

50. Schepers T, Patka P. Treatment of displaced intra-articular calcaneal fractures by ligamentotaxis: current concepts' review. Arch Orthop Trauma Surg 2009;129:1677–83.

51. Elgamel T, Elgamal T, Tanagho A, et al. Temporary external fixation facilitates open reduction and internal fixation of intra-articular calcaneal fractures. Acta Orthop Belg 2013;79:738–41.

52. Yao H, Lu H, Zhao H, et al. Open reduction assisted with an external fixator and internal fixation with calcaneal locking plate for intra-articular calcaneal fractures. Foot Ankle Int 2017;38:1107–14.

53. Duymus T, Mutlu S, Mutlu H, et al. Need for bone grafts in the surgical treatment of displaced intra-articular calcaneal fractures. J Foot Ankle Surg 2017;56:54–8.

54. Lee H, Kang S, Kim J. Surgical treatment of displaced intra-articular fracture of the calcaneus using a Y-plate. J Korean Soc Fract 2002;15:433–8.

55. Illert T, Rammelt S, Drewes T, et al. Stability of locking and non-locking plates in an osteoporotic calcaneal fracture model. Foot Ankle Int 2011;32:307–13.

56. Zang W, Chen E, Xue D, et al. Risk factors for wound complications of closed calcaneal fractures after surgery: a systematic review and meta-analysis. Scand J Trauma Resuscitation Emerg Med 2015;23:18.

57. Wang C-L, Huang S-F, Sun X-S, et al. Abductor digiti minimi muscle flap transfer to prevent wound healing complications after ORIF of calcaneal fractures. Int J Clin Exp Med 2015;8:13001–6.

58. Wong T-W, Sheu H-M, Lee J, et al. Use of tissue meshing technique to facilitate side-to-side closure of large defects. Dermatol Surg 1998;24:1338–41.

Intraoperative Reduction Techniques for Surgical Management of Displaced Intra-Articular Calcaneal Fractures

James M. Cottom, DPM[a],*, Steven M. Douthett, DPM[b],
Kelly K. McConnell, DPM[c]

KEYWORDS

- Calcaneus fracture • Reduction • ORIF • Open reduction internal fixation

KEY POINTS

- Recommendations for surgical repair include displaced intra-articular fractures involving the posterior facet, fracture dislocations, and fractures involving greater than 25% of the calcaneocuboid joint.
- The goal of open reduction internal fixation is restoration of height and length of the calcaneus, anatomic alignment of the posterior facet of the subtalar joint, and realigning the tuber out of varus angulation.
- Lateral extensile, sinus tarsi, closed reduction percutaneous, and closed reduction external fixator methods have all been described for calcaneus repair.

INTRODUCTION

Fractures of the calcaneus are traditionally observed after high-energy trauma. It is essential to perform a full work-up because often concomitant injuries are resultant. Most common concurrent injuries include contralateral calcaneus fractures, ankle fractures, lumbar vertebral fractures, tarsal bone fractures, and fractures of the upper extremity.[1–4] Additionally, patients with such high-energy fractures may suffer abdominal trauma and internal bleeding, reinforcing the need for a full body work-up. The devastating trauma of a calcaneus fracture typically leads to severe edema of the

Disclosures: J.M. Cottom, Consultant to Arthrex.
[a] Florida Orthopedic Foot and Ankle Center Fellowship, 2030 Bee Ridge Suite B, Sarasota, FL 34239, USA; [b] Oregon Medical Group, 600 Country Club Road, Eugene, OR 97401, USA; [c] Coastline Foot and Ankle Center, 800 Liberty Street Southeast, Salem, OR 97302, USA
* Corresponding author.
E-mail address: drcottom@flofac.com

hindfoot and ankle, which may cause soft tissue compromise and fracture blister formation.[1,5] It is essential to rule out compartment syndrome of the hindfoot, which, if left untreated, can result in Volkmann contracture of the foot, necessitating amputation.[6] Literature has shown that prioritizing control of soft tissue edema helps improve incision healing time and decrease wound slough, dehiscence, and subsequent infection.[1,7,8] Ideally, formal surgical repair is performed within 8 hours of injury.[9] Unfortunately, soft tissue compromise and edema often leads to delayed repair. To control edema, bulky jones compression dressings, ice, and elevation are most efficient. Once skin wrinkles return to the lateral heel, it is an indication that edema has receded to allow for incision.[5] Typically, edema is controlled within 7 days to 14 days and surgery may be performed at that time, if necessary. Recommendations for surgical repair include displaced intra-articular fractures involving the posterior facet, fracture dislocations, and fractures involving greater than 25% of the calcaneocuboid joint.[7,8,10]

After careful evaluation of the patient and fracture pattern, the decision to treat the injury surgically versus nonoperatively must be made. Typically, fractures are treated surgically, because the reliability and long-term results of closed reduction and nonoperative treatment are limited and poor. Several factors must be considered when deciding the appropriate surgical approach including a patient's overall health, injury mechanism and fracture pattern, soft tissue integrity, bone quality, and Böhler angle.[11] Restoration of Böhler angle has been shown a predictable measure of long-term success and increased patient outcomes.[12] The goal of open reduction internal fixation is restoration of height and length of the calcaneus, anatomic alignment of the posterior facet of the subtalar joint, and realigning the tuber out of varus angulation.

Literature shows satisfactory results in open reduction internal fixation of displaced intra-articular fractures ranging between 56% and 96%.[2,13] Both lateral and medial approaches have been described, and lateral approaches have been divided into extensile and sinus tarsi incisions. Furthermore, closed reduction and percutaneous or external fixation has been described.

PERCUTANEOUS APPROACH

Closed reduction percutaneous screw fixation was introduced in the early 1980s by Forgon and Zadravecz.[14] In their article, the investigators described placing 2 divergent cancellous screws into the calcaneus after reducing the fracture. Since their original description, several techniques have been described to reduce and fixate calcaneal fractures percutaneously.[15–17] In general, most percutaneous techniques rely on placing a Schanz pin into the posterior tuber to use for traction and manipulation out of varus, along with a lateral stab hole in which a Elevator or other instrumentation may be used to elevate and reduce the posterior facet and, finally, compression of the body of the calcaneus. Percutaneous screws are then inserted to hold reduction. In 2014, Sampath Kumar and colleagues[18] performed a prospective study comparing open reduction internal fixation with minimally invasive reduction and percutaneous fixation in displaced intra-articular calcaneal fractures. These investigators found lower wound complications in the minimally invasive group, with no statistically significant difference in Böhler angle, Gissane angle, and score analysis of Verona. Additionally, the investigators found a quicker return to work time and improved functional outcome scores in the minimally invasive group.[18] The best outcomes have been reported using this approach in patients with minimal comminution and tongue-type fractures and joint-depression fractures, where large tuberosity and sustentaculum fragments may provide support for the screws.[19,20] If surgery is delayed more than 2 weeks, open reduction internal fixation may be more appropriate, because fibrosis between fracture fragments often impedes reduction.[21]

EXTERNAL FIXATION APPROACH

An additional technique for reduction of displaced intra-articular calcaneal fractures that has been well described is use of external fixation.[22–24] This modality can be used in the acute setting to help stabilize calcaneal fractures that necessitate immediate reduction in cases of compartment syndrome, neurovascular injury, or open fractures. Moreover, external fixation can be used in closed reduction of a calcaneal fracture and serve as final formal fixation during healing. The process relies on ligamentotaxis to help realign fracture fragments.

With literature reporting wound breakdown and infection rates up to 33% after use of the traditional lateral extensile incision, there have been numerous recommendations for reducing the risk of soft tissue complications after open reduction internal fixation of calcaneal fractures.[22,24] Use of external fixation, including delta frames, circular frames, and monorails, has been described as an option in preserving the delicate soft tissue envelope in these traumatic injuries.[22–25]

Roukis and colleagues,[22] in 2008, and Kissel and colleagues,[23] in 2011, described use of a delta frame external fixator for reduction of calcaneal fractures. To restore the length and height of the calcaneus, skeletal traction is performed using a Schanz pin through the posterior tuber of the calcaneus, and it is rotated out of varus. With the calcaneus length restored and varus reduced, bicortical Schanz pins may be placed from lateral to medial within the talar neck and distal tibia. Through traction and manual manipulation, the fracture is reduced with the use of intraoperative fluoroscopy, and the carbon fiber rods can be attached to hold reduction of the fracture. After restoration of the gross structure of the calcaneus length and rotation, the posterior facet can be addressed through percutaneous or minimal incisions, if necessary.[22,24]

LATERAL EXTENSILE OPEN REDUCTION INTERNAL FIXATION

The most common approach is the traditional lateral extensile incision. Through use of this incision, the body of the calcaneus is exposed and the posterior facet is easily visualized for reduction. In 2016, Cottom and Baker described a reduction technique using the traditional extensile incision.[26] The patient is positioned in the lateral decubitus position with a tourniquet applied. For best visualization, a lateral extensile approach is used. The vertical arm of the full-thickness incision is placed between the anterior border of the Achilles tendon and the sural nerve, extends to the junction of the plantar and lateral skin, and extends anteriorly to the calcaneocuboid joint with slight dorsal angulation to allow better visualization. The full-thickness flap is mobilized off from the lateral wall of the calcaneus and includes the sural nerve and peroneal tendons. Using a no-touch technique, 2.0-mm Kirschner wires are placed into the distal fibula, talar neck, and navicular to retract the flap, allowing visualization of the lateral calcaneal wall, subtalar joint, and calcaneocuboid joint (**Fig. 1**). After the lateral calcaneal wall is identified, its orientation is marked using electrocautery or skin marker, and it is dissected off the body of the calcaneus. The authors recommend placing this in a moist sponge or saline on the medical instrument stand for later replacement. Next, the posterior facet is identified within the body of the calcaneus. Typically, the posterior facet is depressed and rotated anteriorly. The corresponding posterior facet of the talus is evaluated, and any bony debris is removed from the joint. Next, a lamina spreader may be placed into the body of the calcaneus, with 1 arm oriented directly inferior to the posterior calcaneal facet. Care must be taken to insert the lamina

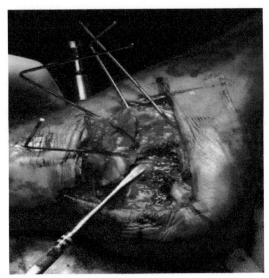

Fig. 1. Kirschner wires placed using no-touch technique. Elevator pointing to posterior facet.

spreader across the entire body of the calcaneus, so the medial aspect of the posterior facet comes into contact with the instrument (**Fig. 2**). The lamina spreader is opened, simultaneously elevating the posterior facet and swinging the posterior tuber out of varus. The spreader is fully expanded, using the talus as a template for proper alignment of the posterior facet (**Fig. 3**). The lamina spreader may be used to dial in reduction of the posterior facet. At this point, lateral and axial calcaneal fluoroscopic images are reviewed for restoration of the calcaneal height and reduction of varus deformity (**Fig. 4**). Any small adjustments in reduction may be performed at this point using a

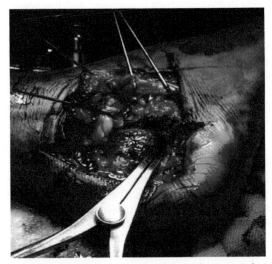

Fig. 2. Lamina spreader placed within the body of the calcaneus, inferior to the posterior facet. Note, the tines are in contact with the medial calcaneal wall.

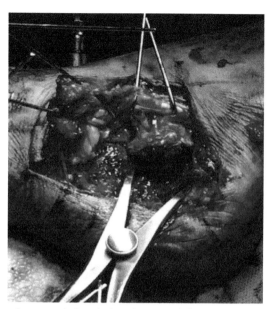

Fig. 3. Lamina spreader expanded, reducing the varus deformity and elevating the posterior facet into anatomic alignment.

Freer elevator. Once the surgeon is satisfied with reduction of the fracture, multiple temporary Kirshner wires are used across any fracture fragments to hold the calcaneus in its reduced alignment. Next, 2 guide wires are inserted from lateral to medial below the posterior facet, into the sustentaculum tali constant fragment. Imaging is used to confirm the guide wires are extra-articular and not violating the medial neurovascular structures, and 4.0-mm cannulated screw fixation is placed. Next, the lamina spreader may be removed, and the body of the calcaneus is filled with bone void filler. The authors typically use an injectable calcium phosphate bone substitute that may be

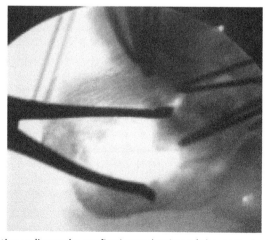

Fig. 4. Intraoperative radiographs confirming reduction of the posterior facet.

molded to fill any remaining bony deficit. Next, the lateral wall is replaced into anatomic position, as marked earlier. A lateral anatomic plate may be applied with a mixture of polyaxial locking and nonlocking screws, in accordance with the fracture pattern. Next, layered closure is performed and a drain is introduced into the proximal incision, evacuating any hematoma. The patient is placed into a bulky jones posterior splint and remains non–weight-bearing until the incision has healed. The authors typically remove the drain in 2 days' to 3-days' time after drainage has subsided.

Cottom and Baker published results using this technique in a radiographic review[26] and found the technique reliably improved Böhler angle, the critical angle of Gissane, and calcaneus varus angles, and all values were statistically significant. Some surgeons advocate for use of a Schanz pin into the posterior tuber for aid in manipulation out of varus; however, the authors have noted multiple instances of poor bone purchase, iatrogenic fracture, and pin site complications (**Fig. 5**).[25] The authors have found that when the tines of a lamina spreader may be inserted under the posterior facet until the medial cortex is felt, when opened, the lamina spreader is efficient at not only elevating the posterior facet but also swinging the posterior tuber in a valgus direction.

Even with meticulous dissection and proper retraction with the no-touch technique, literature reports multiple complications with this incision including hematoma, wound slough, dehiscence, and infection.[7,27–29] Some investigators report the complication rate approaching 33%.[25] To help decrease this wound complication rate, many investigators have advocated using a less-invasive sinus tarsi approach.[1,30]

SINUS TARSI OPEN REDUCTION INTERNAL FIXATION

Sinus tarsi incisional approach to repair calcaneal fractures has been reported in literature.[1,30–32] With lower reported wound complications than the extensile approach, there has been a trend toward this incision in recent times.

The sinus tarsi approach is similar to the lateral subtalar joint arthrodesis approach, with the incision starting approximately 1-cm inferior to the tip of the fibula, extending distally to the base of the fourth metatarsal.[29] After reflecting the extensor digitorum brevis muscle belly dorsally, the surgeon may readily identify the sinus tarsi. This

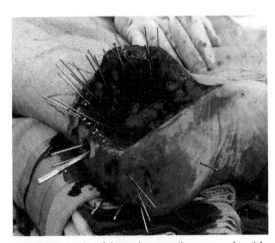

Fig. 5. Intraoperative photograph of lateral extensile approach with reduction using a Schantz pin through the posterior tuber.

incision allows for direct visualization of the posterior facet as well as the anterior process and calcaneocuboid joint. Once exposure is achieved, the surgeon may reduce the varus deformity and realign the posterior facet using a method of preference. The authors' lamina spreader technique described in the extensile approach may be used with this exposure as well. It may be of some help to use a Schanz pin in the posterior tuber to supply traction and rotation to help realign the heel. After reduction is achieved, temporary Kirschner wire fixation is used, and the lamina spreader may be removed. Bone void filler is then used, followed by the final screw and plate construct. With an increased trend toward this approach, multiple plates have been designed for its use.

Weber and colleagues[33] compared sinus tarsi approach to extensile approach in 24 patients. The investigators noted anatomic reduction in both groups, lower operating time, and increased patient reported AOFAS ankle-hindfoot scores with the sinus tarsi approach. The extensile group had a total of 8 complications, including hematoma, sural nerve issues, complex regional pain syndrome, and delayed healing, versus zero complications found within the sinus tarsi group. The investigators noted that 41% of patients within the sinus tarsi approach required screw removal. Similarly, Kline and colleagues[29] performed a retrospective review on 112 calcaneal fractures, comparing the extensile approach to a modified sinus tarsi approach. The investigators reported a 29% wound healing complication rate with the extensile approach versus a 6% wound complication rate in the sinus tarsi approach. The return to operating room rate was 20% in the extensile versus 2% in the minimally invasive group. Patients in the minimally invasive sinus tarsi group reported lower visual analog pain scale levels, improved Foot Function Index score, and increased overall satisfaction.[29]

SUMMARY

This article reviews several techniques for treatment of intra-articular calcaneal fractures. Several factors may lead to the ultimate outcome of a patient's surgery, including fracture morphology, the patient's independent comorbidities, patient expectations, and surgeon experience. Thorough evaluation of these same factors dictates the technique used to best treat this devastating injury. Through less-invasive methods of repair, there has been a trend for improved patient outcomes in recent times. Calcaneal fractures are injuries that can have a dramatic impact on a patient's life; however, surgical reduction and repair using the techniques reviewed in this article can provide satisfactory results.

REFERENCES

1. Mostafa M, El-Adl G, Hassanin E, et al. Surgical treatment of displaced intraarticular calcaneal fracture using a small lateral approach. Strategies Trauma Limb Reconstr 2010;5:87–95.
2. Rowe C, Sakellarides H, Freeman P. Fractures of the os calcis: a long-term follow-up study of one hundred forty-six patients. J Am Med Assoc 1963;184:920.
3. Thordarson D, Krieger L. Operative vs nonoperative treatment of intra-articular fractures of the calcaneus: a prospective randomized trial. Foot Ankle Int 1996; 17:2–9.
4. Van Tetering E, Buckley R. Functional outcome (SF-36) of patients with displaced calcaneal fractures compared to SF-36 normative data. Foot Ankle Int 2004;25: 733–8.
5. Sanders R. Intra-articular fractures of the calcaneus: present state of the art. J Orthop Trauma 1992;6:252–5.

6. Epstein N, Chandran S, Chou L. Current concepts review: intra-articular fractures of the calcaneus. Foot Ankle Int 2012;33:79–86.

7. Bernishcke S, Kramer P. Wound healing complications in closed and open calcaneus fractures. J Orthop Trauma 2004;18:1–6.

8. Howard J, Buckley R, McCormack R, et al. Complications following management of displaced intra-articular calcaneal fractures: a prospective randomized trial comparing open reduction internal fixation with nonoperative management. J Orthop Trauma 2003;17:241–9.

9. Buddecke D, Mandracchia V. Calcaneal fractures. Clin Podiatr Med Surg 1999; 16:769–91.

10. Levin L, Nunley J. The management of soft-tissue problems associated with calcaneal fractures. Clin Orthop 1993;290:151–6.

11. Dooley P, Buckley R, Tough S. Bilateral calcaneal fractures: operative versus nonoperative treatment. Foot Ankle Int 2004;25:47–52.

12. Dhillon M, Bali K, Prabhakar S. Controversies in calcaneus fracture management: a systematic review of the literature. Musculoskelet Surg 2011;95:171–81.

13. Palmer I. The mechanism and treatment of fractures of the calcaneus. J Bone Joint Surg Am 1948;30:2–8.

14. Forgon M, Zadravecz G. Repositioning and retention problems of calcaneus fractures. Aktuelle Traumatol 1983;13:239–46.

15. Pezzoni M, Salvi A, Tassi M, et al. A minimally invasive reduction and synthesis method for calcaneal fractures: the "Brixian Bridge" technique. J Foot Ankle Surg 2009;48:85–8.

16. Forgon M. Closed reduction and percutaneous osteosynthesis: technique and results in 265 calcaneal fractures. In: Tscherne H, Schatzker J, editors. Major fractures of the pilon, the talus, and the calcaneus. Berlin: Springer; 1993. p. 207–13.

17. Aratsu M, Sheehan B, Buckley R. Minimally invasive reduction and fixation of displaced calcaneal fractures: surgical technique and radiographic analysis. Int Orthop 2014;38:539–45.

18. Sampath Kumar V, Marimuthu K, Subramani S, et al. Prospective randomized trial comparing open reduction and internal fixation with minimally invasive reduction and percutaneous fixation in managing displaced intra-articular calcaneal fractures. Int Orthop 2014;38:2505–12.

19. Palmersheim K, Hines B, Olsen B. Calcaneal fractures: update on current treatments. Clin Podiatr Med Surg 2012;29:205–20.

20. Tomesen T, Biert J, Frolke J. Treatment of displaced intra-articular calcaneal fractures with closed reduction and percutaneous screw fixation. J Bone Joint Surg 2011;93(10):920–8.

21. Tennent T, Calder P, Salisbury R, et al. The operative management of displaced intra-articular fractures of the calcaneum: a two-centre study using a defined protocol. Injury 2001;32:491–6.

22. Roukis TS, Wunschel M, Lutz H-P, et al. Treatment of displaced intra-articular calcaneal fractures with triangular tube-to-bar external fixation: long-term clinical follow-up and radiographic analysis. Clin Podiatr Med Surg 2008;25:285–99.

23. Kissel C, Husain Z, Cottom J, et al. Early clinical and radiographic outcomes after treatment of displaced intra-articular calcaneal fractures using a delta-frame external fixator construct. J Foot Ankle Surg 2011;50:135–40.

24. Dayton P, Feilmeier M, Hensley N. Technique for minimally invasive reduction of calcaneal fractures using small bilateral external fixation. J Foot Ankle Surg 2014;53:376–82.

25. Herscovici D, Widmaier J, Scaduto J, et al. Operative treatment of calcaneal fractures in elderly patients. J Bone Joint Surg Am 2005;87:1260–4.
26. Cottom J, Baker J. Restoring the anatomy of calcaneal fractures. A simple technique with radiographic review. Foot Ankle Spec 2016;10:235–9.
27. Al-Mudhaffar M. Wound complications following operative fixation of calcaneal fractures. Injury 2009;31:461–4.
28. Folk J, Starr A, Early J. Early wound complications of operative treatment of calcaneus fractures: an analysis of 190 fractures. J Orthop Trauma 1999;13:369–72.
29. Kline A, Anderson R, Davis W, et al. Minimally invasive technique versus an extensile lateral approach for intra-articular calcaneal fractures. Foot Ankle Int 2013;34:773–80.
30. Femino J, Vaseenon T, Levin D, et al. Modification of the sinus tarsi approach for open reduction and plate fixation of intra-articular calcaneus fractures: the limits of proximal extension based on the vascular anatomy of the lateral calcaneal artery. Iowa Orthop J 2010;30:161–7.
31. Schepers T. The sinus tarsi approach in displaced intra-articular calcaneal fractures: a systematic review. Int Orthop 2011;35:697–703.
32. Gupta A, Ghalambor N, Nihal A, et al. The modified palmar lateral approach for calcaneal fractures: wound healing and postoperative computed tomographic evaluation of fracture reduction. Foot Ankle Int 2003;24:744–53.
33. Weber M, Lehmann O, Sagesser D, et al. Limited open reduction and internal fixation of displaced intra-articular fractures of the calcaneum. J Bone Joint Surg Br 2008;90:1608–16.

Arthroscopic and Endoscopic Management of Common Complications After Displaced Intra-Articular Calcaneal Fractures

Tun-Hing Lui, MBBS (HK), FRCS (Edin), FHKAM, FHKCOS[a],*,
Xiao-hua Pan, MD[b,c,d], Yu Pan, MD[b,c,d]

KEYWORDS

- Calcaneal fractures • Complications • Arthroscopy • Endoscopy • Tendoscopy

KEY POINTS

- There is great potential in managing the lateral complications of calcaneal fractures arthroscopically and/or endoscopically due to the advances in the foot and ankle arthroscopy and endoscopy.
- Group 1 complications include different impingement syndromes and arthrosis leading to focal hindfoot or ankle pain, which can usually be managed arthroscopically and/or endoscopically.
- Group 2 complications cause functional deficit of the foot and ankle; only selected cases can be managed arthroscopically and/or endoscopically.
- Group 3 complications refer to those causing diffuse and poorly localized pain; surgical treatment is not indicated and may even drastically worsen the patient's condition.
- Careful evaluation and analysis of a patient's problem and detailed surgical planning with appropriate combination of arthroscopic/endoscopic and open procedures are the key to success.

Note: Proofs and reprint requests should be addressed to Dr T.H Lui.
[a] Department of Orthopaedics and Traumatology, North District Hospital, 9 Po Kin Road, Sheung Shui, NT, Hong Kong, China; [b] Guangdong Provincial Engineering Research Center of Wound Repair and Regenerative Medicine, Affiliated Baoan Hospital of Shenzhen, Southern Medical University, The 8th People's Hospital of Shenzhen, Shenzhen, Guangdong 518101, China; [c] Guangdong Provincial Academician Workstation of Wound Repair and Regenerative Medicine, Affiliated Baoan Hospital of Shenzhen, Southern Medical University, The 8th People's Hospital of Shenzhen, Shenzhen, Guangdong 518101, China; [d] Department of Trauma and Orthopedics, Affiliated Baoan Hospital of Shenzhen, Southern Medical University, The 8th People's Hospital of Shenzhen, Shenzhen, Guangdong 518101, China
* Corresponding author.
E-mail address: luithderek@yahoo.co.uk

Clin Podiatr Med Surg 36 (2019) 279–293
https://doi.org/10.1016/j.cpm.2018.10.009
0891-8422/19/© 2018 Elsevier Inc. All rights reserved.

INTRODUCTION

Calcaneal fractures are one the most common foot and ankle fractures and account for 2% of all fractures.[1] The primary fracture line separates the sustentaculum fragment with the tuberosity fragment. The sustentaculum fragment generally remains attached to the talus by the interosseous ligament. The tuberosity fragment displaces superiorly and laterally, resulting in shortening and flattening of the calcaneus. It typically rests in a varus heel position. Impaction of the talar body into the calcaneus can result in lateral cortical bulging.[2]

The potential for disabling malunion after calcaneal fracture is high, whether a patient is treated nonsurgically or surgically, and the malunion can affect the function of the surrounding joints and soft tissues.[2] Sequelae include loss of hindfoot height, heel widening, subfibular (peroneal, calcaneofibular) impingement, calcaneocuboid joint impingement, varus heel, and posttraumatic arthrosis.[2–4] With the flattening of calcaneus, the talus rests in a horizontal, dorsiflexed position and may cause anterior ankle impingement and ankle arthritis.[2,5,6] Loss of hindfoot height leads to shoe-wear problems and leg-length discrepancy. This loss of hindfoot height, together with shortening of the lever arm of the gastrocnemius-soleus complex, can cause a decrease in push-off power.[2,5] Varus hindfoot may cause locked midtarsal joint and stiffness in the foot, increased pressure under the head of the fifth metatarsal, and eccentric loading of the ankle and knee joints.[2,5] Up to 48% of calcaneal fractures have a secondary fracture line extending into the calcaneocuboid joint resulting in an anterolateral fragment. Malunion of this fragment may interfere with calcaneocuboid motion leading to calcaneocuboid joint impingement.[2] Posttraumatic arthrosis may develop in nonsurgically or surgically managed calcaneal fractures with articular incongruity. It can also occur in anatomically reduced fractures in which penetration of the joint by implants or the initial trauma can cause irreversible damage to the articular cartilage.[2,6–8]

Other sources of pain include injury to the sural nerve, intra-articular adhesions, implant impingement, and nonunion.[4,9,10] Injury to the sural nerve may be caused by tension or impingement by the lateral cortical bulge. Iatrogenic sural nerve injury resulting in neuroma formation may be the result of previous surgical treatment.[1] Moreover, approximately 10% of calcaneal fractures develop compartment syndromes of the foot, and, of these, one-half develop clawing of the lesser toes and other foot deformities, including hallux varus, stiffness, and neurovascular dysfunction.[11,12]

Whether the initial calcaneal fracture is managed nonsurgically or surgically, most patients experience improvement in pain and function within 1 year. Thus, early management of calcaneal malunion consists of nonsurgical methods (ie, activity modification, bracing, functional orthoses, and injection) to improve patient comfort and function.[2] When the problems do not resolve with conservative management, different surgical options have been postulated either trying to address all the deformities or concentrating on certain aspects that are most clinically pressing.[3,7,13]

Romash[14] proposed multiplane calcaneal reconstruction with osteotomy to restore the fracture line to the innate form followed by anatomic reconstruction to correct all the deformities associated with the late complications of calcaneal fracture and intended to achieve union through subtalar fusion, because the calcaneus acts as a pedestal or platform that supports the talus at the proper height, inducing the appropriate talar declination angle, which is important to ankle motion.[5] This multiplane reconstruction is technically demanding and sometimes it is overdone because not all the deformities are symptomatic at the same time.[6] Huang and colleagues[15] proposed a simpler technique of subtalar fusion with sliding corrective osteotomy of posterior calcaneal tubercle. Although the sliding corrective osteotomy does not provide much improvement to the talus declination angle, it is suitable for those patients with a banana-shaped calcaneus malunion.[15] For those patients who have significant anterior ankle pain caused by loss of heel height and tibiotalar impingement, subtalar distraction bone-block arthrodesis may be performed to restore hindfoot alignment and talocalcaneal relationship.[15] Myerson and Quill,[16] however, as well as Flemister and colleagues[7] cautioned against aggressive attempts to restore heel height because this may lead to hindfoot varus.

Some investigators proposed surgical treatments based on radiological classification of malunion. Stephens and Sanders type I malunions was treated with a lateral wall exostectomy and peroneal tenolysis; type II malunions with a lateral wall exostectomy, peroneal tenolysis, and subtalar arthrodesis; and type III malunions with a lateral wall exostectomy, peroneal tenolysis, subtalar block arthrodesis, and calcaneal osteotomy.[17,18] This radiological classification, however, may not be in line with a patient's symptoms and clinical findings.

Besides addressing all the deformity during the same operation or operations guided by radiological classification of malunion, another approach is focusing on patient symptoms. Only those pathologies contributing to a patient's symptoms are dealt with surgically.

For the sake of symptom-focused surgical approach, the late complications of calcaneal fractures can be classified according to a patient's symptoms into 3 groups:

Group 1. Those complications causing focal hindfoot or ankle pain
Group 2. Those complications causing functional deficit
Group 3. Those present with diffuse and poorly localized pain

Arthroscopic management of late complications after calcaneal fracture focuses on patient symptoms.[6] With the advance of foot and ankle arthroscopy, tendoscopy, and endoscopy, many of group 1 and some of the group 2 complications after calcaneal fracture can be managed in minimally invasive manner.[19–25] Symptomatic malunion often has multiple components and combinations of different arthroscopic and endoscopic procedures are needed.[6] Identification of the correct sources of symptoms is key to select the most appropriate surgical procedures and ensure that the planned surgical correction specifically addresses the underlying pathology.[2,3,6] Detailed history taking and clinical examination are the most important tools for surgical decision making. Radiologic evaluation of malunions can document heel shortening, talar dorsiflexion, and subtalar or calcaneocuboid arthritis.[8] Radiographic measures should not be the sole determinant for surgical decision making.[2] CT is helpful for planning of the surgery.[6]

GROUP 1 COMPLICATIONS

Pain is the most common problem after calcaneal fractures.[3] The group 1 complications include different impingement syndromes and arthrosis. These can be subdivided according to the location of pain:

1. Lateral heel pain
2. Anterior ankle pain
3. Medial heel pain
4. Posterior ankle pain
5. Posterior heel pain
6. Plantar heel pain

Each location has its own list of sources of pain. Careful examination especially accurate localization of pain and tender spot is the key of success. Different pathologies and locations of pain can coexist.

Lateral Heel Pain

Lateral heel pain can be due to

1. Impingement syndromes, such as peroneal impingement, calcaneofibular impingement, and calcaneocuboid impingement
2. Peroneal tendon problems
3. Synovitis and fibrosis: the anterior, posterior subtalar, calcaneocuboid joints or sinus tarsi
4. Posttraumatic arthrosis: anterior subtalar, posterior subtalar, or calcaneocuboid joint
5. Arthrofibrosis and stiffness: anterior subtalar, posterior subtalar, or calcaneocuboid joint
6. Symptomatic hardware
7. Sural nerve problems

Endoscopic lateral calcaneal ostectomy

Lateral calcaneal cortical bulging can cause calcaneofibular or peroneal impingement syndrome or shoe-wear problems. This is the most frequent pathology causing lateral heel pain after calcaneal fracture. Lateral ostectomy is an important component in surgery for different types of calcaneal malunion.[18] The ostectomy can be performed endoscopically via 2-portal[19] or 3-portal[26] approaches. This procedure starts as posterior subtalar arthroscopy. The soft tissue envelop is stripped from the lateral calcaneal wall to create the working space for endoscopic lateral ostectomy; 2-portal approach is usually sufficient for calcaneofibular impingement. If a patient complains of footwear problem, the 3-portal approach is adopted to achieve a more radical resection of the lateral cortical bulge. Preoperative evaluation with CT scan is helpful to assess the size and location of the lateral calcaneal exostosis, its relations with the lateral malleolus, and the extent of degenerative changes in the subtalar joint.[19] The far lateral degeneration of the subtalar joint as in Stephens and Sanders type I malunion can also be detected and resected arthroscopically.[26]

Peroneal tendoscopy

Peroneal tendon problems, including tenosynovitis, tendinitis, subluxation or dislocation of the tendons, fibrosis, and entrapment of the tendons, are more common in conservative management cases and are caused by impingement by the lateral cortical bulge.[8,27] This may also occur after surgical treatment by Kocher approach, because the tendons are released from their sheaths to provide access to the subtalar joint.[27] Implant irritation is another cause of peroneal tendon problems in previously operated cases. It may present as lateral heel pain with buckling or giving way when walking. Localization of the pain along the peroneal tendons and eliciting pain with passive dorsiflexion and resistance to eversion of the hindfoot can confirm peroneal tendons as the source of pain.[16] Loss of active eversion may be the result of peroneal impingement, tendon scarring or frank dislocation.[2] Peroneal tenogram can be considered as preoperative investigation to detect presence and site of blockade within tendon sheath.[28,29] The underlying cause should be treated and endoscopic lateral calcaneal ostectomy is indicated if the tendon problem is due to impingement by the cortical bulge. Peroneal tendoscopy can then be performed for tenolysis, decompression, débridement, repair, synovectomy, and retinaculum reconstruction.[2,19,25,30,31] Tendoscopy portals can be placed along the peroneal tendons and at the proximal and distal ends of the pathology.

Arthroscopic calcaneocuboid decompression

Calcaneocuboid impingement is due to malunion of the anterolateral calcaneal wall fragment, leading to painful loss of motion of the calcaneocuboid joint and increased stress to the adjacent joints.[4] Some investigators have suggested removal of both the residual bone overhang and the lateral fourth of the distal calcaneal facet, because the articulation of this lateral portion with the cuboid is almost always arthritic.[17] This can be performed via calcaneocuboid arthroscopy (**Fig. 1**).[6] After removal of the overhang, the joint is examined for any synovitis or cartilage damage. The extent of joint resection is titrated by the extent of cartilage damage.[6] Impingement and arthrosis of the calcaneocuboid joint can be the ends of a spectrum of severity. Sometimes, it is difficult to judge whether bone resection or arthrodesis is more appropriate. Moreover, resection of the lateral portion of the joint may increase the load and accelerate the degeneration process of the remaining damaged cartilage. Whenever in doubt, the lesser operative procedure is preferable to the irreversible procedure.[32]

Arthroscopic synovectomy

Posttraumatic synovitis of the anterior/posterior subtalar and/or calcaneocuboid joint is one of the causes of lateral heel pain after calcaneal fracture.[33] The posterior subtalar and calcaneocuboid joints can be approached via the respective arthroscopy.[20,24] The anterior subtalar joint synovitis is a commonly missed diagnosis. It usually presents with sinus tarsi pain and sometimes also medial heel pain around the sustentaculum tali. Tenderness can be elicited by deep palpation of the soft spot between the talonavicular and calcaneocuboid joints and pointing posteromedially.[6] The lateral part of the joint can be approached via the anterolateral subtalar and dorsolateral midtarsal portals of anterior subtalar arthroscopy.[34,35] Arthroscopic synovectomy, resection of scar tissue, and débridement of damaged cartilage can be performed. Result after arthroscopic débridement of the joints depends on the

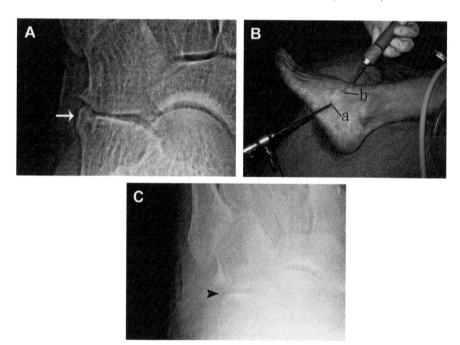

Fig. 1. (A) Radiograph shows calcaneocuboid impingement due to malunion of the anterolateral calcaneal wall fragment (*arrow*). (B) Calcaneocuboid arthroscopy is performed via the lateral (a) and dorsolateral (b) midtarsal portals. (C) Postoperative radiograph shows the impinging bone spur is resected (*arrowhead*).

extent of the cartilage damage.[6] If there is extensive cartilage damage, arthroscopic arthrodesis is more appropriate.

Arthroscopic arthrodesis

Posttraumatic arthrosis of the anterior/posterior subtalar and/or calcaneocuboid joint can occur after the calcaneal fracture. Arthroscopic arthrodesis can be performed for those joints with symptomatic arthrosis recalcitrant to conservative management. Arthroscopic in situ subtalar arthrodesis is indicated in cases of symptomatic subtalar arthrosis without significant hindfoot malalignment.[2,26,35,36] The initial management of calcaneal fracture also affects outcome and may play a role in determining the optimal treatment.[2,37] Subtalar arthrodesis has better functional outcomes and fewer complications if the fracture is initially treated with open reduction and internal fixation.[2,37] Talar dorsiflexion is not contraindicated for in situ arthrodesis if the patients did not have anterior ankle impingement pain.[2,38] This procedure can be performed with either a lateral or posterior approach.[39] The approach selected depends on surgeon preference and the other planned concomitant arthroscopic procedures. The lateral impingement can be worsened by subtalar arthrodesis, which diminishes the height of the talus and calcaneus, especially in case of Sanders type II malunion.[32] The lateral gutter should be carefully examined after arthrodesis and endoscopic lateral ostectomy also should be performed if there is lateral impingement.

In cases of Sanders type III malunion, calcaneal osteotomy is frequently performed in conjunction with the subtalar joint arthrodesis. Another approach is arthroscopic subtalar arthrodesis with closing wedge procedure.[40] The varus heel is corrected by laterally based wedge resection of the subtalar joint during arthrodesis. After the fusion sites were prepared, a lateral wedge of bone of the subtalar joint is resected by an Isham Straight Flute Shannon burr (Vilex, McMinnville, Tennessee) via the subtalar portals.[6] Valgus force is applied to the heel during bone resection to correct the varus heel. Lateral impingement can be worsened after this procedure. The lateral gutter needs to be examined again after the closing wedge procedure, and the lateral gutter is decompressed further if needed.[6]

Calcaneocuboid arthrosis may occur as frequently as subtalar arthrosis does, but it is less frequently symptomatic.[2] Arthroscopic double arthrodesis is indicated if both the calcaneocuboid and subtalar arthrosis are symptomatic.

Arthroscopic triple arthrodesis may be indicated in combined symptomatic calcaneocuboid and subtalar arthrosis with preexisting flatfoot deformity.[2,20] Inclusion of talonavicular joint is also indicated for talonavicular arthrosis, which can be either preexisting or a result of midtarsal stiffness due to hindfoot varus. Deformity of each joint can be corrected with the closing wedge procedure after preparation of the fusion surfaces.[6,40]

Arthroscopic release

Subtalar arthrofibrosis with stiffness is common after surgically managed calcaneal fracture.[6] Inversion stresses are transferred to the ankle joint, especially the lateral ligamentous structures of the ankle, resulting in lateral ankle pain.[17] After surgical release, early postoperative range-of-motion exercise is important to prevent recurrence of hindfoot and ankle stiffness.[2] Open subtalar release is not a good surgical option because early vigorous mobilization exercise is prohibited by the extensive surgical wound.[6] Arthroscopic release of posterior subtalar joint has the advantage of smaller surgical wounds so that immediate vigorous mobilization is allowed.[6,41] The tight lateral capsuloligamentous structures are released via the lateral portals. The soft tissue release is extended beyond the surgical scar in the patients with previous surgery. The interosseous talocalcaneal ligament should be preserved. Occasionally, arthroscopic release of the anterior subtalar joint is also needed. This is performed via the anterolateral subtalar, dorsomedial, and dorsolateral midtarsal portals.[42]

Anterior Ankle Pain

Pain over the anterior ankle or midfoot dorsum can be due to

1. Anterior ankle impingement
2. Impingement of anterosuperior calcaneal process to the plantar-lateral talar head or navicular bone

   Anterior ankle impingement of the talar neck on the anterior lip of the distal tibia results from loss of calcaneal height and loss of talar declination.[2,5] This problem cannot be managed arthroscopically. Better solution is distraction bone block subtalar arthrodesis to restore talocalcaneal height and talar declination. Distraction arthrodesis should not be performed only according to radiological parameters because clinical studies showed that full correction of the hindfoot alignment parameters is not necessary to obtain a successful clinical result.[7,38] Therefore, distraction arthrodesis is only indicated in the presence of anterior ankle impingement.[6,7,38]

Endoscopic resection of anterosuperior calcaneal process
Occasionally, malunited anterosuperior calcaneal process with elongation of the process or unhealed fragment at this region can impinge on the plantar lateral side of the talar head or navicular bone.[6] The patient complains of local swelling, deep pain, and tenderness at that region and limited foot inversion and the diagnosis can be confirmed by oblique radiograph of the foot.[6] Endoscopic excision of the elongated or unhealed anterosuperior calcaneal process is indicated if conservative treatment failed to relieve the symptoms.[43–45] The working (dorsolateral midtarsal) portal is at the junction between the talonavicular and calcaneocuboid joints. The lateral midtarsal portal at the plantar-lateral corner of the calcaneocuboid joint is the viewing portal.[20] After decompression of the potential space between the talonavicular and calcaneocuboid joints, the plantar lateral part of the talar head and navicular bone is examined for any chondral lesion. Arthroscopic débridement and microfracture is performed if the lesion is present.

Medial Heel Pain

1. Tarsal tunnel syndrome
2. Flexor hallucis longus (FHL) tendon problems
3. Synovitis at medial gutter of anterior subtalar joint
4. Arthrofibrosis at medial gutter of anterior subtalar joint

Endoscopic tarsal tunnel release
In some cases of calcaneal fracture, displacement of the tuberosity resulting in valgus deformity may place tension along the tibial nerve as it traverses the tarsal tunnel.[2] Occasionally, tibial nerve problems are caused by direct bony impingement.[2] The patient may report vague medial foot pain and/or heel pain and the Tinel sign may be noted posterior to the medial malleolus.[2] Endoscopic tarsal tunnel release is indicated if conservative treatment is failed to relieve the symptoms.[46] This provides a better environment for nerve recovery. Preoperative CT is essential to exclude any bony impingement of the nerve. Open tarsal tunnel release and resection of the impinging bone is indicated if the tarsal tunnel syndrome is caused by bony impingement.

Zone 2 flexor hallucis longus tendoscopy
Zone 2 FHL tendon refers to the part of the tendon from fibro-osseous tunnel of posterior talus to the master knot of Henry.[47] Because of the proximity of the FHL tendon to the

medial surface of the calcaneus, fractures and malunions in this region may result in scarring and/or tethering of the FHL tendon under sustentaculum tali.[2] This is Lui type 1A posttraumatic fibrous adhesions, where the adhered tendon does not turn within the fibrous sheath.[48] The patient may present with local medial heel pain, limited motion, and/or cock-up deformity of the hallux. Pain can be reproduced by passive dorsiflexion of the hallux.[2] Preoperative CT is needed to study any bony impingement of the FHL tendon in the osseofibrous tunnel under the sustentaculum tali by bone fragment or malunion.[49] Zone 2 FHL tendoscopy is performed via the posteromedial and plantar portal.[47] Tenolysis should be started at the bone-tendon interface and proceed to the tendon-fibrous sheath interface.[48] Release of the tendon from the fibrous tendon sheath should be performed carefully because perforation of the tendon sheath may damage the medial plantar nerve, which locates at the plantar medial side of the fibro-osseous tunnel.[50,51]

Medial subtalar arthroscopy

Calcaneal fracture involving the anterior/middle facet can cause synovitis, chondral lesion, and/or arthrofibrosis of the anterior subtalar joint. If the pathologies locate at the medial side of the joint, the patient experiences medial heel pain. These conditions cannot be dealt with by the anterior subtalar arthroscopy, and medial subtalar arthroscopy should be performed via the medial midtarsal and medial tarsal canal portals (**Fig. 2**).[23,33,52] The portals are interchangeable as the viewing and working portals. Arthroscopic synovectomy can be performed via these portals. If there is arthrofibrosis of the joint causing painful eversion of the foot, arthroscopic resection of the fibrous tissue and stripping of the medial capsule from the subtentaculum tali are performed (**Fig. 3**).[53] The capsule should not be stripped dorsally because the perforating vessels to the medial talus may be damaged.[33]

The fibrous adhesion between the talar head and the spring ligament is also lysed and the spring ligament is preserved to maintain the stability of the talocalcaneonavicular joint.[53] After release, the plantar medial part of the talar head and the sustenaculum tali are examined for any chondral lesion (**Fig. 4**). Débridement and microfracture of the chondral lesion are performed if chondral lesion is present.

Posterior Ankle Pain

Posterior ankle pain can be due to

1. Posterior ankle impingement by malunion of joint depressed–type calcaneal fracture
2. Fibrosis or tenosynovitis of the FHL tendon posterior to the ankle joint
3. Fibrosis of distal FHL muscle

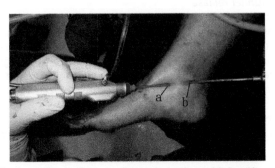

Fig. 2. Medial subtalar arthroscopy is performed via the medial midtarsal (a) and medial tarsal canal (b) portals.

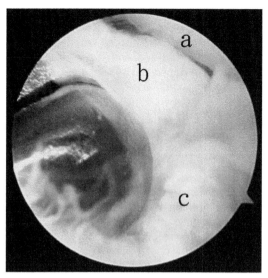

Fig. 3. Arthroscopic view shows stripping of the medial capsule from the subtentaculum tali: a, talar head; b, subtentaculum tali; and c, fibrotic medial capsule.

Endoscopic posterior ankle decompression

A calcaneal bone spike can be formed just posterior to the depressed posterior calcaneal facet in cases of malunion of the joint depressed–type calcaneal fracture.[6,22] Posterior ankle impingement pain can occur when the thick scar tissue at the posterior ankle is pinched between the posterior tibial lip and the bone spike during ankle plantarflexion. The bony impediment and the scar tissue can be resected via 2-portal posterior ankle endoscopy.[54] The portals should be placed above the posterosuperior calcaneal tubercle to approach the posterior ankle.[6] The posterior joint line of the

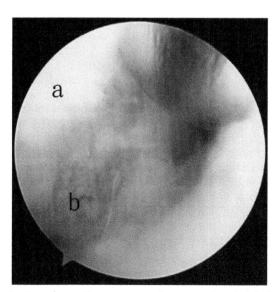

Fig. 4. Arthroscopic view shows the presence of an oseochondral lesion at the plantar medial side of the talar head: a, talar head and b, osteochondral lesion.

posterior subtalar joint usually cannot be seen even after resection of the scar tissue because the posterior calcaneal facet is depressed and the view is obscured by the bone spike. The bone spike is resected with an arthroscopic burr with caution not to damage the posterior facet cartilage and the cartilage of the posterior talar dome. The adequacy of bone resection can be confirmed arthroscopically and fluoroscopically with passive ankle plantarflexion.

Endoscopic synovectomy and tenolysis of zone 1 flexor hallucis longus tendon
Zone 1 FHL tendon locates posterior to the ankle and tenosynovitis and adhesions can occur after calcaneal fracture. This can be approached via posterior portals and endoscopic synovectomy and tenolysis can be performed.[47]

Endoscopic adhesiolysis of flexor hallucis longus muscle
Fibrosis of distal FHL muscle can be a result of subclinical compartment syndrome of the distal deep posterior compartment of the leg. This can occur after calcaneal fracture because of the communication between calcaneal compartment and the distal deep posterior compartment of the leg.[55] It presents with deep posterior ankle pain with local tenderness just above the posterior ankle joint line. Endoscopic adhesiolysis of the muscle can be performed via the posterior portals.[56,57] The release is performed from lateral edge of the muscle and proceed medially. Immediate postoperative mobilization of the ankle and hallux are important for prevention of recurrence of adhesions.

Posterior Heel Pain
Posterior heel pain can occur after malunion of tongue-type calcaneal fracture.[58] It is due to the secondary Haglund deformity impinging on the Achilles tendon.[58] This bony prominence can be resected by endoscopic calcaneoplasty.[59,60] This procedure can be performed with a patient in supine or prone position, depending on the concomitant procedures planned. Sometimes, the scar tissue between the bone and the Achilles tendon should be resected before the Achilles insertion can be clearly seen.[6]

Plantar Heel Pain
Plantar heel pain after calcaneal fracture usually cannot be dealt with endoscopically. It can be due to

1. Plantar exostosis
2. Injury to the heel pad
3. Tarsal tunnel syndrome

Plantar pain after calcaneal fracture is most commonly secondary to plantar exostosis.[5] Palpation may reveal regions of plantar bony prominence that correlate with a patient's pain.[2] A standing lateral radiograph is the best investigation to confirm the exostosis impinging on the plantar heel pad. Symptomatic plantar exostosis can be resected percutaneous with an Isham Straight Flute Shannon burr.[61]

Plantar heel pain may also be caused by injury to the soft tissues that attach the heel pad to the calcaneus or to the heel pad itself. Injury to this region results in diffuse tenderness on the plantar aspect of the calcaneal tuberosity. The surgeon may observe atrophy of the heel pad, which may be a result of the original injury.[2] Surgery is contraindicated for posttraumatic heel pad atrophy.

GROUP 2 COMPLICATIONS

Th group 2 complications cause functional deficit. For example, loss of calcaneal length may cause weakness of the ankle plantar flexion with easy fatigue of the calf muscle. Other problems include foot and toes deformities as a result of compartment syndrome of the foot or tendon adhesions around the calcaneus. Most of the complications of this group request open surgical procedures, for example, corrective osteotomy, open soft tissue release, or tendon transfer.[33] In cases of flexible hallux deformity due to adhesion of FHL tendon under sustentaculum tali, zone 2 FHL tendoscopy and tenolysis can be performed. In cases of rigid hallux valgus or hallux varus deformity as a result of foot compartment syndrome, arthroscopic arthrodesis of the first metatarsophalangeal joint can be performed.[12,62,63]

GROUP 3 COMPLICATIONS

The group 3 complications include complex regional pain syndrome and heel pad atrophy.[5] These complications usually cannot be managed surgically. Surgical treatment may drastically worsen a patient's condition.

FORMULATING AND EXECUTING THE OPERATIVE PLAN: PORTAL ECONOMY, PATIENT POSITIONING, AND CONTRADICTING REHABILITATION PROGRAMS

Post–calcaneal fracture residual pain likely results from a mix of intra-articular and extra-articular disorders. It is necessary to perform a combination of procedures, both intra-articular and extra-articular, to relieve the pain.[4]

After identifying all the sources of a patient's symptoms, the surgeon can list out the operative procedures needed. The procedures are then grouped according to the following criteria:

1. Procedures for the most clinically pressing symptoms have priority
2. Procedures are grouped according to those requiring supine, prone, and lateral patient positioning. This allows proper arrangement of the sequence of procedures and avoids unnecessary change in patient position during the operation.
3. Procedures requiring different postoperative rehabilitation plan should be grouped separately and performed in different operation settings.
4. Procedures that share the portals can be grouped and performed during the same operation

Economy of Portal Usage

Careful planning of portal placement can reduce the number of portals needed because many portals can be shared for different arthroscopic and endoscopic procedures:

1. Posterolateral portal: zone 1 FHL tendoscopy; posterior subtalar arthroscopy; endoscopic calcaneoplasty; and endoscopic posterior ankle decompression
2. Posteromedial portal: zone1 and zone 2 FHL tendoscopy; endoscopic calcaneoplasty; and endoscopic posterior ankle decompression
3. Anterolateral subtalar portal: posterior subtalar arthroscopy and anterior subtalar arthroscopy
4. Dorsolateral midtarsal portal: talonavicular arthroscopy; anterior subtalar arthroscopy; calcaneocuboid arthroscopy; and endoscopic resection of anterosuperior calcaneal process

For example, a patient with symptomatic secondary posterior ankle impingement and calcaneofibular impingement can have the following operation planning. Posterior ankle decompression is performed via posteromedial and posterolateral portals with the patient in prone position. Endoscopic lateral calcaneal osteotomy and peroneal

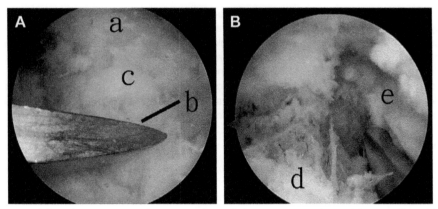

Fig. 5. (A) Endoscopic view shows resection of the posterior calcaneal bone spike with an osteotome. (B) Endoscopic lateral calcaneal ostectomy via the posterior portals: a, distal tibia; b, posterior calcaneal bone spike; c, talar dome; d, calcaneus; and e, lateral malleolus.

tendon release can be performed with the patient in lateral or prone position. The lateral decompression and peroneal tendon release are usually performed via the lateral portals. The procedures also can be done, however, via the posterior portals. Therefore, the final surgical plan is endoscopic posterior ankle decompression, lateral calcaneal ostectomy, and peroneal tendon release via the posteromedial and postero-lateral portals with the patient in prone position (**Fig. 5**).[64] This surgical plan saves the unnecessary lateral portals and intraoperative change of patient position.

RESULTS

Except for surgical technique description, only small case reports/series are available. What has been published is generally favorable, with resolution of pain and meaningful improvement in function, and this parallels the authors' experience.[4,6,19,22,26,36,41,44,48,64]

SUMMARY

Arthroscopic and endoscopic management of late complications after calcaneal fractures is a symptom-focused approach. Careful evaluation and analysis of patient problems and detailed surgical planning with appropriate combination of arthroscopic and open procedures are the key to success. There is no large-scale long-term study to demonstrate the efficacy, and safety of this minimally invasive approach and the procedures should be used with caution. Finally, most of these procedures are technically demanding and should be reserved for the foot and ankle surgeons experienced in complex arthroscopy, endoscopy, and tendoscopy procedures about the hindfoot.

REFERENCES

1. Yeap EJ, Rao J, Pan CH, et al. Is arthroscopic assisted percutaneous screw fixation as good as open reduction and internal fixation for the treatment of displaced intra-articular calcaneal fractures? Foot Ankle Surg 2016;22:164–9.

2. Banerjee R, Saltzman C, Anderson RB, et al. Management of calcaneal malunion. J Am Acad Orthop Surg 2011;19:27–36.
3. Li Y, Bao RH, Jiang ZQ, et al. Complications in operative fixation of calcaneal fractures. Pak J Med Sci 2016;32:857–62.
4. Yoshimura I, Ichimura R, Kanazawa K, et al. Simultaneous use of lateral calcaneal ostectomy and subtalar arthroscopic debridement for residual pain after a calcaneal fracture. J Foot Ankle Surg 2015;54:37–40.
5. Young KW, Lee KT, Lee YK, et al. Calcaneal reconstruction for the late complication of calcaneus fracture. Orthopedics 2011;34:e634–8.
6. Lui TH, Chan KB. Arthroscopic management of late complications of calcaneal fractures. Knee Surg Sports Traumatol Arthrosc 2013;21:1293–9.
7. Flemister AS, Infante AF, Sanders RW, et al. Subtalar arthrodesis for complications of intra-articular calcaneal fractures. Foot Ankle Int 2000;21:392–9.
8. Lim EVA, Leung JPF. Complications of intraarticular calcaneal fractures. Clin Orthop Relat Res 2001;391:7–16.
9. Kumar N. Non-union of calcaneum : a rare complication of calcaneal fracture – a case report with brief review of literature. J Clin Orthop Trauma 2015;6:187–9.
10. Wajdi B, Rebai MA, Baya W, et al. Pseudarthrosis of the calcaneus: advantages of regenerative medicine in the management of a rare entity a case report and review of literature. Open Orthop J 2018;12:141–6.
11. Myerson M, Manoli A. Compartment syndromes of the foot after calcaneal fractures. Clin Orthop Relat Res 1993;290:142–50.
12. Dayton P, Haulard JP. Hallux varus as complication of foot compartment syndrome. J Foot Ankle Surg 2011;50:504–6.
13. Reddy V, Fukuda T, Ptaszek AJ. Calcaneal malunion and nonunion. Foot Ankle Clin N Am 2007;12:125–35.
14. Romash MM. Reconstructive osteotomy of the calcaneus with subtalar arthrodesis for malunited calcaneal fractures. Clin Orthop Relat Res 1993;290:157–67.
15. Huang PJ, Fu YC, Cheng YM, et al. Subtalar arthrodesis for late sequelae of calcaneal fractures: fusion in situ versus fusion with sliding corrective osteotomy. Foot Ankle Int 1999;20:166–70.
16. Myerson MS, Quill GE Jr. Late complications of fractures of calcaneus. J Bone Joint Surg Am 1993;75:331–41.
17. Clare MP, Lee WE III, Sanders RW. Intermediate to long-term results of a treatment protocol for calcaneal fracture malunions. J Bone Joint Surg Am 2005;87:963–73.
18. Stephens HM, Sanders R. Calcaneal malunions: results of a prognostic computed tomography classification system. Foot Ankle Int 1996;17:395–401.
19. Bauer T, Deranlot J, Hardy PH. Endoscopic treatment of calcaneo-fibular impingement. Knee Surg Sports Traumatol Arthrosc 2011;19:131–6.
20. Lui TH. New technique of arthroscopic triple arthrodesis. Arthroscopy 2006;22:464.e1-e5.
21. Lui TH. Current concepts: foot and ankle arthroscopy and endoscopy: indications of new techniques. Arthroscopy 2007;23:889–902.
22. Lui TH. Posterior ankle impingement syndrome caused by malunion of joint depressed type calcaneal fracture. Knee Surg Sports Traumatol Arthrosc 2008;16:687–9.
23. Mekhail AO, Heck BE, Ebraheim NA, et al. Arthroscopy of the subtalar joint: establishing a medial portal. Foot Ankle Int 1995;16:427–32.
24. Oloff L, Schulhofer SD, Fanton G, et al. Arthroscopy of the calcaneocuboid and talonavicular joints. J Foot Ankle Surg 1996;35:101–8.

25. van Dijk CN, Kort N. Tendoscopy of the peroneal tendons. Arthroscopy 1998;14: 471–8.

26. Lui TH. Endoscopic lateral calcaneal ostectomy for calcaneofibular impingement. Arch Orthop Trauma Surg 2007;127:265–7.

27. Bahari Kashani M, Kachooei AR, Ebrahimi H, et al. Comparative study of peroneal tenosynovitis as the complication of intraarticular calcaneal fracture in surgically and non-surgically treated patients. Iran Red Crescent Med J 2013;15: e11378.

28. Bhattacharyya A, Raman R. Mal-united fracture of calcaneum treated with lateral decompression. Mymensingh Med J 2013;22:148–56.

29. Chen W, Li X, Su Y, et al. Peroneal tenography to evaluate lateral hindfoot pain after calcaneal fracture. Foot Ankle Int 2011;32:789–95.

30. Lui TH. Endoscopic peroneal retinaculum reconstruction. Knee Surg Sports Traumatol Arthrosc 2006;14:478–81.

31. Lui TH. Endoscopic management of recalcitrant retrofibular pain without peroneal tendon subluxation or dislocation. Arch Orthop Trauma Surg 2012;132:357–61.

32. Connolly JF. Persistent heel pain twenty years after calcaneal fracture and triple arthrodesis relieved by lateral decompression. J Trauma 1987;27:809–10.

33. Lui TH. Medial subtalar arthroscopy. Foot Ankle Int 2012;33:1018–23.

34. Lui TH. Clinical tips: anterior subtalar (talocalcaneonavicular) arthroscopy. Foot Ankle Int 2008;29:94–6.

35. Lui TH, Chan KB, Chan LK. Portal safety and efficacy of anterior subtalar arthroscopy: a cadaveric study. Knee Surg Sports Traumatol Arthrosc 2010;18:233–7.

36. Mi K, Liu P, Liu W, et al. Arthroscopic subtalar arthrodesis for malunion of calcaneal fractures. Zhongguo Xiu Fu Chong Jian Wai Ke Za Zhi 2010;24:875–7.

37. Radnay CS, Clare MP, Sanders RW. Subtalar fusion after displaced intra-articular calcaneal fractures: does initial operative treatment matter? J Bone Joint Surg Am 2009;91:541–6.

38. Chandler JT, Anderson RB, Davis WH, et al. Results of in situ subtalar arthrodesis for late sequelae of calcaneus fractures. Foot Ankle Int 1999;20:18–24.

39. Perez Carro L, Golanó P, Vega J. Arthroscopic subtalar arthrodesis: the posterior approach in the prone position. Arthroscopy 2007;23:445.e1-e4.

40. Lui TH. Case report: correction of neglected club foot deformity by arthroscopic assisted triple arthrodesis. Arch Orthop Trauma Surg 2010;130:1007–11.

41. Lui TH. Arthroscopic subtalar release of post-traumatic subtalar stiffness. Arthroscopy 2006;22:1364.e1-e4.

42. Lui TH. Arthroscopic release of lateral half of the talocalcaneonavicular joint. Arthrosc Tech 2016;5(6):e1471–4.

43. Lui TH. Arthroscopic resection of the calcaneonavicular coalition or the "too-long" anterior process of the calcaneus. Arthroscopy 2006;22:903.e1-e4.

44. Lui TH. Endoscopic excision of symptomatic nonunion of anterior calcaneal process. J Foot Ankle Surg 2011;50:476–9.

45. Lui TH. Arthroscopic resection of too-long anterior process (TLAP) of the calcaneus. Arthrosc Tech 2016;5(5):e1179–83.

46. Day FN 3rd, Naples JJ. Tarsal tunnel syndrome: an endoscopic approach with 4- to 28-month follow-up. J Foot Ankle Surg 1994;33(3):244–8.

47. Lui TH. Flexor hallucis longus tendoscopy: a technical note. Knee Surg Sports Traumatol Arthrosc 2009;17:107–10.

48. Lui TH. Arthroscopic and endoscopic management of posttraumatic hindfoot stiffness. Indian J Orthop 2018;52:304–8.

49. Komiya K, Terada N. Entrapment of the flexor hallucis longus tendon by direct impalement in the osseofibrous tunnel under the sustentaculum tali: an extremely rare complication of a calcaneal fracture: a case report. JBJS Case Connect 2014;4:e100.
50. Lui TH, Chan KB, Chan LK. Zone 2 flexor hallucis longus tendoscopy: a cadaveric study. Foot Ankle Int 2009;30:447–51.
51. Lui TH, Chan KB, Chan LK. Cadaveric study of zone 2 flexor hallucis longus tendon sheath. Arthroscopy 2010;26:808–12.
52. Lui TH, Chan LK, Chan KB. Medial subtalar arthroscopy: a cadaveric study of the tarsal canal portal. Knee Surg Sports Traumatol Arthrosc 2013;21:1279–82.
53. Lui TH. Arthroscopic capsular release of the talocalcaneonavicular joint. Arthrosc Tech 2016;5:e1305–9.
54. van Dijk CN, Scholten PE, Krips R. A 2-portal endoscopic approach for diagnosis and treatment of posterior ankle pathology. Arthroscopy 2000;16:871–6.
55. Bayer JH, Davies AP, Darrah C, et al. Calcaneal compartment syndrome after tibial fractures. Foot Ankle Int 2001;22:120–2.
56. Lui TH. Endoscopic adhesiolysis of flexor hallucis longus muscle. Arthrosc Tech 2017;6:e325–9.
57. Lui TH. Endoscopic adhesiolysis of the flexor hallucis longus muscle. Foot Ankle Spec 2014;7:492–4.
58. Jung HG, Yoo MJ, Kim MH. Late sequelae of secondary Haglund's deformity after malunion of tongue type calcaneal fracture: report of two cases. Foot Ankle Int 2002;23:1014–7.
59. Lui TH. Technique tip: reattachment of the Achilles tendon after endoscopic calcaneoplasty. Foot Ankle Int 2007;28:742–5.
60. van Dijk CN, van Dyk E, Scholten PE, et al. Endoscopic calcaneoplasty. Am J Sports Med 2001;29:185–9.
61. Lui TH. Technical tip: percutaneous bone shaving and ulcer endoscopy to manage abnormal pressure point of the sole. Foot 2014;24:190–4.
62. Lui TH. Arthroscopic arthrodesis of the first metatarsophalangeal joint in hallux valgus deformity. Arthrosc Tech 2017;6:e1481–7.
63. Lui TH. Arthroscopic first metatarsophalangeal arthrodesis for repair of fixed hallux varus deformity. J Foot Ankle Surg 2015;54:1127–31.
64. Lui TH. Endoscopic management of calcaneofibular impingement and posterior ankle impingement syndrome secondary to malunion of joint depressed type calcaneal fracture. Arthrosc Tech 2018;7:e71–6.

Primary or Secondary Subtalar Arthrodesis and Revision of Calcaneal Nonunion with Minimally Invasive Rigid Internal Nail Fixation for Treatment of Displaced Intra-Articular Calcaneal Fractures

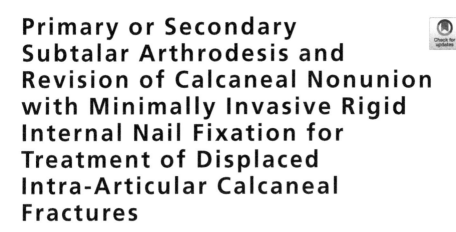

Didier Fuentes-Viejo, MD, PhD[a], Gabriel Cellarier, MD[a], Philien Lauer[b],
Patrick Simon, MD, PhD[c], Thomas Mittlmeier, MD, PhD[b],*

KEYWORDS

- Sequelae after calcaneal fractures • Posttraumatic osteoarthritis of the subtalar joint
- Minimally invasive approach • Primary subtalar joint arthrodesis
- Distraction subtalar joint arthrodesis • Complications

KEY POINTS

- Subtalar joint arthrodesis represents a valuable principle of treating displaced calcaneal fractures as a primary or secondary intervention strategy.
- Subtalar joint arthrodesis with an interlocking nail can be performed via minimally invasive approaches.
- Subtalar joint arthrodesis with an interlocking nail offers angular stability without inherent risk of secondary loss of correction.
- Subtalar joint arthrodesis with an interlocking nail can be applied as a salvage solution for subtalar joint nonunion.

Disclosure: T. Mittlmeier and P. Simon are coinventors of the Calcanail and receive royalties from FH Orthopaedics, Heimsbrunn, France. The other authors have nothing to disclose.
[a] Institut Pied & Cheville, Centre Hospitalier d'Agen, Route de Villeneuve sur Lot, Saint-Esprit, Agen F-47923 Cedex 9, France; [b] Department of Trauma, Hand and Reconstructive Surgery, Rostock University Medical Center, Schillingallee 35, Rostock D-18057, Germany; [c] 14 rue Victor Hugo, Lyon F 69002, France
* Corresponding author.
E-mail address: Thomas.mittlmeier@med.uni-rostock.de

Clin Podiatr Med Surg 36 (2019) 295–306
https://doi.org/10.1016/j.cpm.2018.10.010

INTRODUCTION

Subtalar joint arthrodesis represents a powerful tool for addressing a variety of indications of congenital, degenerative, and posttraumatic pathologies.[1-6] From the technical aspect, in situ and distraction bone block arthrodesis can be separated into primary and secondary subtalar joint arthrodesis. Primary subtalar joint arthrodesis had been successfully applied in cases of severely comminuted displaced intraarticular calcaneal fractures (DIACFs), where the probability of restoring the integrity of the articular surfaces is limited.[7,8] The reasons for secondary subtalar fusion after DIACFs were formulated by Myerson and Quill,[9] who described a loss of heel height greater than 8 mm and anterior ankle impingement due to an abnormal talar declination angle as the decisive parameters for restoring hindfoot geometry.[6,9] Some investigators questioned geometric or radiographic alterations as the relevant conditions for indicating distraction arthrodesis and promoted the relevance of clinical assessment of pain and range of motion at the ankle joint, speaking in favor of or against an in situ arthrodesis[10]; an in situ arthrodesis hardly allows for restoration of hindfoot anatomy and biomechanics[6] or addresses the typical pathologies after DIACFs with shortening and widening of the hindfoot and associated peroneal tendon impingement or subfibular abutment.[6,11,12] Despite the observation that less deformity and malalignment, as in the situation after open reduction with internal fixation of DIACFs, is correlated with better functional outcomes and fewer complications after subtalar joint arthrodesis,[13] there has not been any convincing proof that an in situ arthrodesis had less complications and a higher union rate than a bone block distraction arthrodesis.[14]

Independent of the surgical variants of in situ and distraction arthrodesis, the application of screws represents the most frequently applied technique for surgical fixation in subtalar joint arthrodesis. Most clinical reports about the outcome parameters of subtalar bone block distraction arthrodesis focused on the clinical results—the functional assessment as gait analysis and successful union—with only occasional notes on secondary malalignment or loss of correction until final healing.[3-5,11,12,15-17] Therefore, the frequency of partial backing out of the screws and implant loosening and final loss of reduction is not yet evaluated.

To the best of the authors' knowledge, there has not been any report about angular stable fixation in subtalar fusion, until now. Calcaneal interlocking nailing (Calcanail, FH Orthopedics, Mulhouse, France, and Chicago, Illinois) was introduced in 2012 as a novel minimally invasive concept in the treatment portfolio of calcaneal fractures, with promising clinical results.[18,19] A high primary stability of calcaneal interlocking nailing had proved comparable to interlocking plating in a cadaver model of a standardized DIACF during dynamic testing.[20,21] The same implant concept with a larger nail diameter and extended nail lengths is available for any variant of subtalar joint arthrodesis. As such, it was the goal of the authors' study to introduce into this novel technique applied in the calcaneal fracture or postfracture situation and to display some of the first short-term clinical results.

BIOMECHANICS OF SUBTALAR JOINT ARTHRODESIS TECHNIQUES

One to 3 fully threaded positioning screws inserted from the talar neck into the calcaneus or vice versa from the calcaneal tuberosity into the center of the talar body represent the most frequently applied clinical mode for fixation of a subtalar joint arthrodesis.[1,2,4,6,11-13,15,16] The use of standard compression screws seems more susceptible for loss of reduction than fully threaded screws because the compression effect might get lost early after surgery before osseous healing occurs. This may occur, in particular, in cases of compromised bone quality, which refers to both the bone block and the adjacent osseous structures or in primary subtalar arthrodesis after a DIACF, where a substantial defect has to be bridged by the screws.[7,8] Under laboratory conditions, headless compression screws might be advantageous compared with standard compression screws, where a compression arthrodesis technique is feasible.[21,22] Screws with divergent directions are considered less sensitive than parallel screws against various types of instability.[23,24] Two parallel screws in the typical position should be augmented by a third screw inserted from the lateral plantar calcaneal rim into the talar neck.[22] Despite that there is no report about the in vitro performance of the implant until now, an interlocking nail is generally regarded as one of the most stable constructs, where the implant position is near the mechanical axis of the corresponding bone. The few studies where the in vitro performance of intramedullary interlocking nails had been studied in a calcaneal fracture model confirmed that the nail was as strong as or even stronger than conventional plates or interlocking plates.[20,21] The locking screws of the Calcanail are tapered near the crew head, which is conical and buried into the lateral calcaneal wall. Together with the oval cross-section of the corresponding nail's locking holes, a backing out of the screws is prevented and an angular stable interlocking mode is created (**Fig. 1**).

INSTRUMENTATION AND SURGICAL TECHNIQUE OF SUBTALAR JOINT ARTHRODESIS VIA INTERLOCKING NAILING

The instrument tray of the Calcanail contains both the instruments for stabilization of a calcaneal fracture and subtalar joint arthrodesis (**Fig. 2**). Whereas the implant for the fracture situation has a diameter of 10 mm with duplicate interlocking, the standard implant diameter for subtalar joint arthrodesis has a diameter of 12 mm and is available in 3 lengths, with 3 interlocking options (see **Fig. 2**A). Cannulated interlocking screws have identical diameters for both indications. In general, 3 interlocking screws are recommended for subtalar arthrodesis to maximally enhance the stability of the construct. The implant should be positioned centrally within the calcaneus and in the anterior and lateral third of the talar body to respect the physiologic hindfoot alignment and to avoid any interference with the lateral ankle during proximal interlocking (see **Fig. 2**A, B).

The surgical procedure can be performed either in a prone, lazy lateral, or lateral decubitus position (**Figs. 3** and **4**). The latter might be performed on top of a sterile

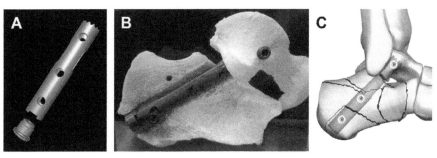

Fig. 1. The Calcanail implant comes in 1 diameter of 12 mm and 3 lengths of 65 mm, 75 mm, and 85 mm (*A*). An end cap is available to prevent fibrous ingrowth into the inner structure of the nail in case of later need for implant removal. Plastic model displaying the preferred position of the nail for subtalar joint arthrodesis (*B*). Schematic drawing of final nail position (*lateral view*) (*C*). (*Courtesy of* FH Orthopedics, Chicago, IL.)

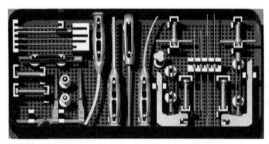

Fig. 2. Calcanail instrument tray. (*Courtesy of* FH Orthopedics, Chicago, IL.)

draped fluoroscopic receiver (see **Fig. 3**). In cases of need for additional procedures as a lateral calcaneal osteotomy due to widening of the calcaneus with lateral calcaneal wall abutment or peroneal tendon impingement, a posterior soft tissue release and/or Achilles tendon lengthening a posterolateral approach is preferable. Mostly, a skin incision of 6-cm length is sufficient. Furthermore, it allows for a large-scale inspection of the subtalar joint from lateral to medial and the sinus tarsi anteriorly if a distraction device is used intraoperatively. Preparation should be kept strictly lateral from the flexor hallucis longus tendon to protect the neurovascular bundle, which runs medially from the tendon. Otherwise, a sinus tarsi approach with 3-cm to 4-cm length is adequate for débridement of the talar cartilage in cases of primary arthrodesis after a DIACF (ie, Sanders type IV fracture pattern[25]) or in posttraumatic osteoarthritis after a conservative treatment of a DIACF to remove the remnants of cartilage from the calcaneus and talus and to débride any subchondral bone sclerosis (**Fig. 5**). Chisels, curettes, or motorized burrs may be applied for this task (see **Fig. 5B**). Depending on previous surgical interventions, the surgical approach might be dictated by the need for implant removal, such as a calcaneal plate originally placed via the extended lateral approach.

It is of utmost importance to restore the anatomic position of the hindfoot. Therefore, large Caspar distraction or compression devices with 3.2-mm pins are elements

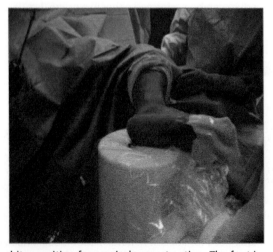

Fig. 3. Lateral decubitus position for surgical reconstruction. The foot is position directly on the fluoroscope, which had been draped before.

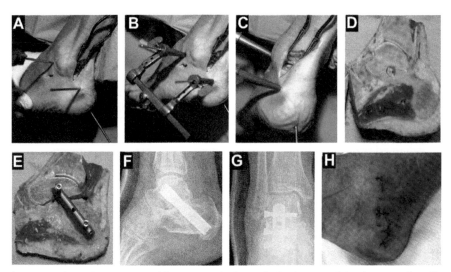

Fig. 4. Lazy lateral or prone position are used when a limited posterolateral approach to the subtalar joint and a limited sinus tarsi approach are needed. The 2 pins for the large distractor had been inserted near to the lateral talar process and the calcaneal tuberosity to support the correction of hindfoot malalignment and calcaneal shortening. The posterior guide pin within the calcaneal tuberosity demonstrates the posterior approach for nail insertion (*A*). The large distractor has been mounted for a stepwise correction of the deformity (lateral [*B*] and posterior [*C*] views). Sagittal central saw cut of a cadaver hindfoot (*D*) demonstrating the correct position of the implant within the bones (*E*). Particular attention should be paid to the adequate choice of the nail length, avoiding any protrusion from the calcaneal tuberosity and soft tissue interference. Postoperative lateral (*F*) and anterior-posterior (*G*) radiographs after nail insertion in 2 planes demonstrating the central position in the anterior-posterior view and the position of the nail tip within the anterior third of the talar body on the lateral view. Postoperative lateral picture of the hindfoot displaying the minimally invasive approaches (*H*).

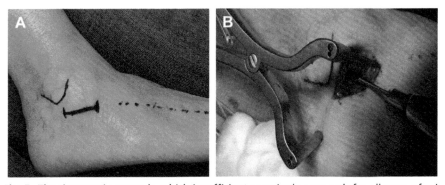

Fig. 5. The sinus tarsi approach, which is sufficient as a single approach for all cases of primary arthrodesis after calcaneal fracture and those cases of limited need for height restoration of the hindfoot to remove the remnants of cartilage and eventually insert a bone graft (*A*). The large distractor should be positioned without interference with the surgical tools needed for removal of the cartilage remnants and the subchondral bone sclerosis with a motorized burr (*B*).

of the Calcanail instrumentation tray to allow for restoration of the anatomic talocalcaneal alignment (see **Figs. 4** and **5; Fig. 6**). The reduction instruments should be kept in place until the implant has been securely fixed to avoid any inadvertent intraoperative loss of reduction. In particular, any hindfoot varus malalignment should be strictly avoided. The long guide pin for reaming of the bone canal for the implant is inserted next after reduction from the chamfered central posterior side of the calcaneal tuberosity (see **Fig. 6; Fig. 7**). Its position should be checked carefully via fluoroscopy in 2 planes because it defines the terminal position of the implant. The 12-mm motorized trephine is inserted via the guide pin. The reaming process up to the talar dome should be performed under repetitive fluoroscopic control to avoid any perforation into the ankle joint (see **Fig. 7**). The hollow reamer creates a longitudinal autologous bone graft, which can be used as an autogenous bone graft to fill the gaps between the realigned talus and calcaneus or to fill the implant itself. In cases of a sclerotic talar bone, a drill with identical diameter as the final implant may be used, in addition, to prepare the bone canal (see **Fig. 7**D, E). Length measurement presents the next step, where it is important that the chosen nail length does not implicate any posterior protrusion of the implant or an intraoperative talar neck fracture. The selected implant is fixed to a handle and inserted manually into its final position in the bone channel under fluoroscopic control (**Fig. 8**). A targeting device is fixed to the nail holding handle for insertion of the interlocking screws. Drill sleeves demarcate the area for the corresponding stab incisions on the lateral side of the hindfoot. Usually, 2 interlocking screws are fixed within the calcaneus and 1 within the talus. First, the 1.6-mm Kirschner wires from the instrumentation set are inserted that allow for the length measurement before they are over-drilled with a 3.7-mm cannulated drill. During placement of the interlocking screws, fluoroscopy guides the surgeon to bury the conical compression screw head under the lateral calcaneal and talar bone such that the surface is flush without any protruding screw segments. Doing so optimizes the angular stability of the nail construct. Furthermore, screws that are too long are proud medially and cause interference with the long flexor tendons and the medial neurovascular bundle and should be avoided. In contrast to conventional screw arthrodesis techniques, the structural bone graft, if indicated, should be inserted and impacted after the final positioning of the nail implant to avoid any potential destruction of the graft due to the large size implant. After the insertion of the interlocking screws, the dimensions of the planned graft size can be re-evaluated. Using the posterolateral approach, 2 tricortical autologous iliac crest grafts can be impacted along the medial and lateral aspects of the centrally positioned nail.[26] An end cap closes the hollow nail and helps avoid fibrous ingrowth into the end of the implant.

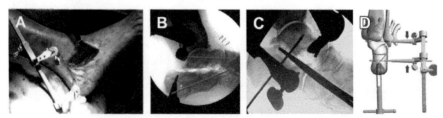

Fig. 6. The large distractor has been mounted to restore the hindfoot height (*A*). A second compressive device might be helpful to restore the talocalcaneal divergence and axes (*B*). The guide pin for manual reaming has been inserted and should carefully be checked via fluoroscopy for an optimal position before reaming (*C*). A compression device may be helpful to obtain a correct talo-calcaneal alignment before insertion of the nail (*D*).

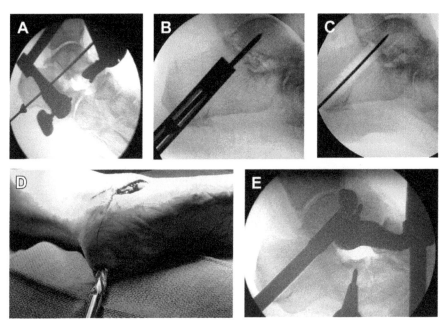

Fig. 7. The reaming sequence for the implant canal is demonstrated on lateral intraoperative fluoroscopic images with the guide wire (*A*), reamer (*B*), and final implant path (*C*) occurring within the calcaneus and talus, taking care not to perforate into the ankle joint. In cases of very sclerotic bone, a motorized reamer or cannulated drill can alleviate the controlled preparation of the bone canal, as demonstrated in the intraoperative photograph (*D*) and lateral fluoroscopic image (*E*).

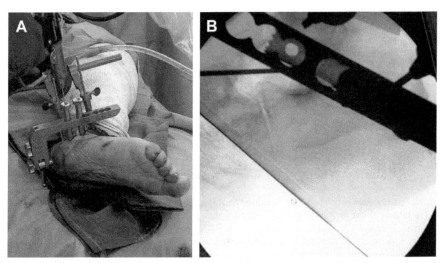

Fig. 8. Intraoperative photograph (*A*) and lateral fluoroscopic view (*B*) demonstrating the wire sleeves through the aiming jig that has been mounted to the nail.

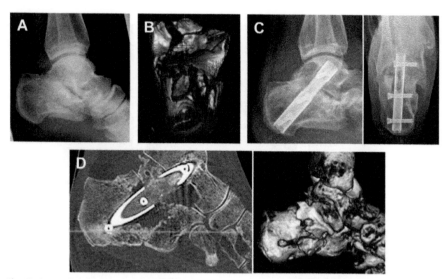

Fig. 9. Lateral radiograph (*A*) and 3-D CT scan image (*B*) of a comminuted calcaneal fracture (Sanders type IIIAB with severe destruction of the lateral and central elements) where a primary fusion was indicated. Lateral (*left*) and axial (*right*) postoperative radiographs of the hindfoot (*C*) and CT scan images (*D*) 4 months after primary fusion demonstrating progressive osseous healing.

Postoperatively, the patient's leg is put in a lower leg splint for a few days, which is replaced then by a lower leg orthosis for a total of 5 weeks to 6 weeks. Partial weight bearing is begun depending on the uneventful soft tissue healing and recommended for a total of 6 weeks with a gradual transfer to full weight bearing within 2 weeks.

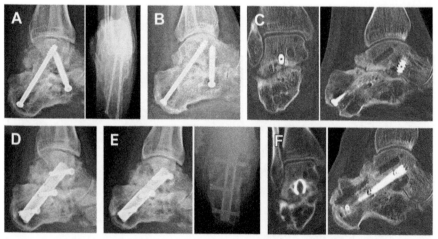

Fig. 10. Distraction bone block arthrodesis of the subtalar joint with screws is demonstrated in the lateral (*left*) and axial (*right*) radiographs (*A*). This resulted in the development of a painful nonunion 9 months after surgery as demonstrated on the lateral heel radiograph (*B*) and coronar (*left*) and sagittal (*right*) CT image reconstructions (*C*). Lateral radiograph 2 weeks following revision (*D*), lateral (*left*) and long axial (*right*) views 6 months after revision (*E*). The coronar (*left*) and sagittal (*right*) reconstructions of the CT scans 6 months after revision document the osseous integration of the autologous bone graft (*F*).

Exercises of the ankle and midfoot joints are started under physiotherapeutic control from the immediate postoperative period.

CLINICAL RESULTS

A subtalar joint arthrodesis using the interlocking nail was performed in 12 patients (median age 55 years) from December 2013 to November 2017. The indication was a DIACF (1 case; **Fig. 9**), a posttraumatic osteoarthritis after a DIACF (6 cases; **Fig. 10**), and a revision arthrodesis after nonunion after screw arthrodesis (5 cases; **Fig. 11**). After a median follow-up of 14 months, a delay union had been observed

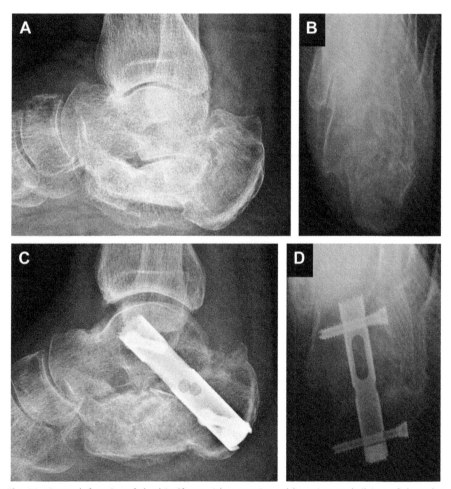

Fig. 11. Gross deformity of the hindfoot with posterior subluxation and tilting of the talus demonstrated on lateral (A) and axial (B) heel views due to substantial loss of calcaneal height and substance with inherent impossibility of the 74-year-old patient to bear weight on the right hindfoot 30 years after conservative treatment of a DIACF. Soft tissue scarring did not allow for a complete restoration of the hindfoot geometry. Despite this, the patient benefitted substantially from the elimination of the anterior tibiotalar impingement and gain in hindfoot stability as demonstrated on the postoperative lateral (C) and axial (D) heel radiographs.

in 1 case, which did not necessitate surgical revision. Loss of correction compared with the postsurgical state was not observed in a single case.

DISCUSSION

Subtalar joint arthrodesis after calcaneal fractures represents a valuable option for primary and secondary indications.[6,7,13,27] Patients after primary arthrodesis in cases of a DIACF did not prove to have functionally inferior outcomes compared with patients with primary open reconstruction.[7,8,25,27] In cases of secondary subtalar distraction bone block arthrodesis, large-diameter fully threaded screws (6.5 mm and/or 7.3 mm) represent the most frequently used fixation tools to maintain the reconstruction of the hindfoot.[3,6] The outcome after isolated subtalar joint arthrodesis is generally considered successful, with union rates ranging from 84% to 100%,[4,6,11] whereas substantially lower union rates, approximately 71%, are observed after subtalar revision arthrodesis.[4] Apart from functional outcome scores and an increase in heel height compared with the preoperative situation, in screw arthrodesis techniques there is only scattered information about the terminal loss of correction after union. Some investigators reported about varus or valgus malunions (up to 7%), graft subsidence, and symptomatic implants that might hint at gradual implant migration during the osseous healing process.[6] An angular stable interlocking nail with 3 interlocking options compatible with various minimally invasive surgical approaches represents a more rigid fixation mode than the screw technique. Therefore, the former might better maintain the result of surgical reconstruction until osseous healing independent from the choice of the bone graft material or any additional implant.[17,28] The first pilot series discussed in this article seems to support the notion that the interlocking maintained the geometric reconstruction until osseous healing occurred. This was also true in cases of revision subtalar arthrodesis. The novel fixation technique in combination with minimally invasive approaches also may be preferable in patients with compromised bone quality and concomitant diseases that delay osseous healing, such as diabetes mellitus, and provides high primary stability in situations where patients cannot adhere to a partial weight-bearing regime.

REFERENCES

1. DiDomenico LA, Butto DN. Subtalar joint arthrodesis for elective and posttraumatic foot and ankle deformities. Clin Podiatr Med Surg 2017;34:327–38.
2. Davies MB, Rosenfeld PF, Stavrou P, et al. A comprehensive review of subtalar arthrodesis. Foot Ankle Int 2007;28:295–7.
3. Deorio JK, Leaseburg JT, Shapiro SA. Subtalar distraction arthrodesis through a posterior approach. Foot Ankle Int 2008;29:1189–94.
4. Easley ME, Trnka HJ, Schon LC, et al. Isolated subtalar arthrodesis. J Bone Joint Surg Am 2000;82:613–24.
5. Schepers T. The subtalar distraction bone block arthrodesis following the late complications of calcaneal fractures: a systematic review. Foot (Edinb) 2013; 23:39–44.
6. Espinosa N, Vacas E. Subtalar distraction arthrodesis. Foot Ankle Clin 2018;23: 485–98.
7. Schepers T. The primary arthrodesis for severly comminuted intra-articular fractures of the calcaneus: a systematic review. Foot Ankle Surg 2012;18:84–8.
8. Holm JT, Laxson SE, Schubert JM. Primary subtalar joint arthrodesis for comminuted fractures of the calcaneus. J Foot Ankle Surg 2015;54:61–5.

9. Myerson M, Quill GE Jr. Late complications of fractures of the calcaneus. J Bone Joint Surg Am 1993;74:331–41.

10. Chandler JT, Bonar SK, Anderson RB, et al. Results of in situ subtalar arthrodesis for late sequelae of calcaneus fractures. Foot Ankle Int 1999;20:18–24.

11. Rammelt S, Grass R, Zawadski T, et al. Foot function after subtalar distraction bone-block arthrodesis. A prospective study. J Bone Joint Surg Br 2004;86: 659–68.

12. Baravarian B. Block distraction arthrodesis for the treatment of failed calcaneal fractures. Clin Podiatr Med Surg 2004;21:241–50.

13. Radnay CS, Clare MP, Sanders RW. Subtalar fusion after displaced intra-articular calcaneal fractures: does initial operative treatment matter? Surgical technique. J Bone Joint Surg Am 2010;92(Suppl 1 Pt 1):32–43.

14. Dingemans SA, Backes M, Goslings JC, et al. Predictors of nonunion and infectious complications in patients with posttraumatic subtalar arthrodesis. J Orthop Trauma 2016;30:e331–5.

15. Fuhrmann RA, Pillukat T. Subtalar arthrodesis. Oper Orthop Traumatol 2016;28: 177–92.

16. Haskell A, Pfeiff C, Mann R. Subtalar joint arthrodesis using a single lag screw. Foot Ankle Int 2004;25:774–7.

17. Chiang CC, Tzeng YH, Lin CF, et al. Subtalar distraction arthrodesis using fresh-frozen allogeneic femoral head augmented with local autograft. Foot Ankle Int 2013;34:550–6.

18. Goldzak M, Mittlmeier T, Simon P. Locked nailing for the treatment of displaced articular fractures of the calcaneus: description of a new procedure with Calca-nail. Eur J Orthop Surg Traumatol 2012;22:345–9.

19. Simon P, Goldzak M, Eschler A, et al. Reduction and internal fixation of displaced intra-articular calcaneal fractures with a locking nail: a prospective study of sixty-nine cases. Int Orthop 2015;39:2061–7.

20. Reinhardt S, Martin H, Ulmar B, et al. Interlocking nailing versus interlocking plating in intraarticular calcaneal fractures: a biomechanical study. Foot Ankle Int 2016;37:891–7.

21. Dingemans SA, Sintenie FW, deJong VM, et al. Fixation methods for calcaneal fractures: a systematic review of biomechanical studies. J Foot Ankle Surg 2018;57:116–22.

22. Matsumoto T, Glisson RR, Reidl M, et al. Compressive force with 2-screw and 3-screw subtalar joint arthrodesis with headless compression screws. Foot Ankle Int 2016;37:1357–63.

23. Eichinger M, Schmölz W, Brunner A, et al. Subtalar arthrodesis stabilization with screws in an angulated configuration is superior to the parallel disposition: a biomechanical study. Int Orthop 2015;79:2275–80.

24. Jastifer JR, Alrafeek S, Howard P, et al. Biomechanical evaluation of strength and stiffness of subtalar arthrodesis joint arthrodesis screw constructs. Foot Ankle Int 2016;37:419–26.

25. Sanders R, Vaupel ZM, Erdogan M, et al. Operative treatment of displaced intra-articular calcaneal fractures: long-term (10-20 years) results in 108 patients using a prognostic CT classification. J Orthop Trauma 2014;28:551–63.

26. Saß M, Rotter R, Mittlmeier T. Minimally invasive internal fixation of calcaneal fractures or subtalar joint arthrodesis using the Calcanail®. Oper Orthop Traumatol 2018. [Epub ahead of print].

27. Dingemans SA, Meijer ST, Backes M, et al. Outcome following osteosynthesis versus primary arthrodesis of calcaneal fractures: a cross-sectional cohort study. Injury 2017;48:2336–41.
28. Wiewiorski M, Barg A, Horisberger M, et al. Revision subtalar joint fusion with a porous metal spacer and an intramedullary nail: a case report. J Foot Ankle Surg 2015;54:709–12.

Management of Calcaneal Fracture Malunion with Bone Block Distraction Arthrodesis

A Systematic Review and Meta-Analysis

Mitchell J. Thompson, DPM[a], Thomas S. Roukis, DPM, PhD[b,*]

KEYWORDS

- Calcaneal • Malunion • Arthrodesis • Subtalar joint • Bone block • Revision
- Surgery

KEY POINTS

- Subtalar bone block arthrodesis has been described as a revision surgery to restore hindfoot alignment and calcaneal height in calcaneal malunion.
- Limited data are available concerning complications of subtalar bone block arthrodesis after failed conservative or surgical treatment of calcaneal fractures.
- Restoring calcaneal height, width, and length while maintaining neutral hindfoot alignment is the priority in calcaneal reconstruction surgery.
- It is vital for a surgeon to understand complications and union rates for bone block arthrodesis surgery when used for calcaneal malunion.
- One of the most severe complications in calcaneal fractures is a malunion.

INTRODUCTION

Fractures of the calcaneus have long been considered one of the most difficult fractures to treat.[1] Although calcaneal fractures account for only 2% of all fractures, they can account for up to 70% of all fractures in the tarsal bones.[2] Approximately

---

Disclosure Statement: Dr T.S. Roukis is a consultant for DePuy Synthes, FH ORTHO, Integra, and Novastep. Owns intellectual property rights with Crossroads Extremity, Novastep, and Stryker. Serves on the Clinical Research of Foot & Ankle and has received grant/research funding from Gundersen Health System Medical Foundation.
^a Podiatric Medicine and Surgery Resident, Gundersen Medical Foundation, Mail Stop CO3-006A, 1900 South Avenue, La Crosse, WI 54601, USA; ^b Orthopaedic Center, Gundersen Healthcare System, Mail Stop CO2-006, 1900 South Avenue, La Crosse, WI 54601, USA
* Corresponding author.
E-mail address: tsroukis@gundersenhealth.org

Clin Podiatr Med Surg 36 (2019) 307–321
https://doi.org/10.1016/j.cpm.2018.10.011
0891-8422/19/© 2018 Elsevier Inc. All rights reserved.

80% of these fractures have are intra-articular.[3] The literature agrees on the principles of restoring calcaneal morphology, specifically returning the calcaneus to proper height, length, and width with the additional goal of restoring the articular surfaces of the subtalar joint.[4] It has been shown that as little as 2 mm of displacement along the articular surface of the subtalar joint can greatly alter the contact pressure leading to further complications.[5] Unfortunately, debate still exists regarding the best way to treat displaced intra-articular calcaneal fractures (DIACF).[3,5] These methods include conservative cares, minimally invasive approaches, open reduction and internal fixation, and external fixation.[3] Surgical management of DIACF involves a steep and unforgiving learning curve that requires a high level of specialized surgical skills.[3] Conservative cares in the setting of a DIACF, as well as inadequate surgical reduction, can lead to significant complications.[6] These complications vary widely from soft tissue, nerve, and bone-related complications, with the most significant being deep wounding and infection, chronic pain syndromes, posttraumatic arthritis, and mal/nonunion of the calcaneus.[1,3] Yu and colleagues[7] identified calcaneal fracture malunion to be 8 times more common than nonunion following open reduction and internal fixation.[7] One major complication of a calcaneal malunion is anterior ankle impingement secondary to reduction in calcaneal height and concomitant decrease in the talar declination. Other significant complications include lateral calcaneal wall deformation leading to impingement and pain about the Sural nerve and peroneal tendons, as well as varus hindfoot alignment with posttraumatic subtalar joint arthritis that, over time, can cause ankle and midtarsal joint compensatory wear.[6] All told, calcaneal fracture malunion results in a significant altered quality of life secondary to persistent pain and reduced function.

Multiple surgical procedures have been described as salvage procedures for calcaneal fracture malunion, and range from exostectomy of the lateral wall or of the anterior tibia/talus, peroneal tendon repair, and Sural neurolysis/resection if there has been damage caused by the lateral wall exostosis, calcaneal realignment osteotomy to reduce any hindfoot malalignment, and subtalar joint arthrodesis with bone block interposition to correct loss in calcaneal height, structural varus deformity, and resect the arthritic subtalar joint surfaces.[6,8] In 1988, Carr and colleagues[9] were the first to describe the subtalar distraction arthrodesis with the use of a contoured bone block for calcaneal malunion with the goals defined as restoration of calcaneal height and width to allow for improved ankle range of motion.[9] The specific surgical technique consisted of a posterior-lateral incision to gain visualization of the posterior subtalar joint. Subsequent preparation of this joint was followed by insertion of an autogenous iliac crest cortico-cancellous bone block that was tailored to defect size to correct the deformities present. Internal fixation across the subtalar joint was performed with solid 6.5-mm screws.[9] As one might expect with revision surgery, there also comes the risk of complications. When attempting arthrodesis, the risk of nonunion and malunion are of greatest concern. In fact, it has been described that nonunion rates are higher with bone block distraction than with in situ subtalar joint arthrodesis.[10] To the authors' knowledge, there has been only 1 systematic review performed on subtalar bone block distraction arthrodesis for revisional calcaneal surgery.[8] In 2012, Schepers[8] performed a systematic review reporting primarily on union rate, subjective patient satisfaction scores, and time to return to work, along with mention of published complications. Since the review by Schepers,[8] additional studies have been published with more contemporary bone grafting, internal fixation methods, larger numbers of patients, and longer-term follow-up. The purpose of our study was to perform an updated systematic review of the available literature starting from the publication of Carr and colleagues[9] and quantitative synthesis of this information. The aim being to report on complications seen and severity of these complications along with union incidence following subtalar bone block distraction arthrodesis exclusively for the treatment of calcaneal malunion following treatment of DIACF.

PATIENTS AND METHODS

We undertook an extensive search of 3 electronic databases, including Cochrane Database of Systematic Review (http://www.cochrane.org/reviews/; last accessed July 15, 2018), PubMed (https://www.ncbi.nlm.nih.gov/pubmed?otool=wiulltlib; last accessed July 25, 2018), and Ovid SP (http://www.ovid.com/site/index.jsp; last accessed July 7, 2018). Google scholar (https://scholar.google.com/; last accessed July 30, 2018) was also used as a general search engine to identify any additional literature not included in the aforementioned databases. These Internet-based databases were searched from April through July of 2018. There were no date or language restrictions. Articles not written in English were translated by the first author using the Internet-based translator Google translate (https://translate.google.com/, last accessed July 11, 2018.) The languages requiring translation into English were German, Korean, French, and Chinese.

An all-inclusive search was performed using key words "bone block," "arthrodesis," "subtalar joint," "fusion" with Boolean operators "AND" and "OR" to also include "calcaneal malunion" and "calcaneus fracture." After reviewing the article titles for relevance, the appropriate abstracts were then reviewed and finally the full article was obtained for review, which included a complete review of the publication's references to search for any missed data. Textbook chapters, technique guides, and review articles were also searched for any additional pertinent information.

Inclusion criteria stated each study must have a total number of procedures at final follow-up of $\geq$10 surgeries involving patients $\geq$18 years of age undergoing a subtalar joint arthrodesis using a bone block distraction technique specifically for calcaneal malunion. In publications in which multiple different techniques of arthrodesis were performed, the results had to be reported in a way to obtain only results pertinent to the bone block arthrodesis. Similarly, in journal articles where indications for the bone block arthrodesis consisted of more than calcaneal malunion, the results needed to be reported in such a way as to ascertain only the calcaneal malunion data. The studies used in our review must have reported on complications and these needed to have been reported in full, allowing the authors to differentiate between minor and major complications, as well as between soft tissue and bone complications. Further, if multiple indications for surgery were used, complication reporting had to allow us to determine the complications directly related to the calcaneal malunion. We considered minor complications to include superficial wounding, hardware irritation/removal, neuropraxia, and exostoses. We considered major complications to include radiographically apparent/symptomatic nonunion, symptomatic malunion, revision surgeries for arthrodesis or calcaneal osteotomies, deep infections requiring surgical intervention, surgical neurolysis or unresolved/permanent nerve injury, and chronic pain syndromes.

STATISTICAL ANALYSIS

We undertook a quantitative synthesis of our pooled cohort data using the double arcsine transformation as described by Barendregt and colleagues.[11] Heterogeneity was analyzed by performing calculations for Cochran's Q test, which is calculated through the squared deviations contributed from each study. The total degrees of freedom (n − 1) used for the calculations was set at 15, as we had 16 total studies in our review. *P* values were also calculated for the soft tissue versus bone complications to determine the statistical significance of our data. Odds ratios were unable to be calculated because of heterogeneity of the reporting of complications in the 16 studies, and with our variables of, number of procedures above and below 15 and dates of publication before and after 2005, we were unable to develop individualized odds ratios for each study, making an overall odds ratio unattainable. Fisher's exact test was ultimately used to compare the competing variables of publication year and number of procedures with the distinction of soft tissue and bone complications (**Tables 1** and **2**).

RESULTS

Our Internet-based search identified 388 articles that were considered potentially relevant to our systematic review. After initial title review, the number of articles eligible for review was 97. Following abstract and then full article review, 16 studies ultimately met our inclusion criteria and were included (**Fig. 1**). Seven articles did undergo translation for full review (3 Chinese, 2 French, 1 German, and 1 Korean), but only the 1 Chinese article ultimately met our inclusion criteria.

Table 3 includes the specific information included in our systematic review and quantitative synthesis. The 16 included studies yielded 278 total procedures in patients with a weighted mean age of 42.6 ± 6.86 years (range: 28.7–56.0 years) with a mean weighted follow-up time, for the studies that reported it, of 40.3 ± 25.38 months (range: 7.7–108.0 months). The mean weighted union rate for all 278 procedures was 95.78% ± 0.0425% (range: 89.47%–100%; 95% confidence interval: 92.35%–98.41%). The surgeons performing these procedures were consistent with their approach either being a lateral extensile or posterior-lateral approach. Lateral incision was described in 9 publications, resulting in 148 (53%) total procedures. The posterior-lateral approach was used in 130 (47%) of the procedures and discussed in 8 publications. One study performed by Baravarian[12] used both approaches, with the lateral approach being performed only in patients who had previous open reduction and internal fixation that required hardware removal.[12] Hardware necessitating removal at time of surgery was reported in 4 of the studies for a total of 23 (8.3%) procedures.

Complications were separated into 1 of 4 categories with our predetermined inclusion criteria. These categories were minor bone or soft tissue and major bone or soft tissue complications. There were 45 (16.2%) minor soft tissue complications and 37 (13.3%) minor bone complications. Minor soft tissue complications were recognized

Table 1				
Number of soft tissue complications				
		Year of Publication		
Procedures	No. of Complications	≥2005	<2005	Total
>15 Procedures	No. of complications	1	6	7
	Column %	3.13	31.58	
	Row %	14.29	85.71	
≤15 Procedures	No. of complications	31	13	44
	Column %	96.88	68.42	
	Row %	70.45	29.55	
Total	No. of complications	32	19	51

P = .007934.

Table 2 Number of bone complications		Year of Publication		
Procedures	No. of Complications	≥2005	<2005	Total
>15 Procedures	No. of complications	0	16	16
	Column %	0.00	43.24	
	Row %	0.00	100.00	
≤15 Procedures	No. of complications	18	21	39
	Column %	100.00	56.76	
	Row %	46.15	53.85	
Total	No. of complications	18	37	55

$P = .000476$.

as temporary paresthesia and superficial soft tissue infection not requiring surgery. Minor bone complications consisted of lateral calcaneal wall exostosis requiring shoe gear modification or resection and hardware removal. Major complications reported for all 278 procedures were 6 (2.2%) major soft tissue complications and 18 (6.5%) major bone complications. Major soft tissue complications were reported as deep infection requiring surgical intervention, complete nerve loss resulting in muscle dysfunction or decreased limb function, and complex regional pain syndromes. Major bone complications consisted of nonunion requiring surgery or malunion requiring osteotomies to correct hindfoot structure. The overall incidence of complications was 38% (106/278), keeping in mind this is reported for all procedures and not per patient, as many patients could have had more than 1 complication. This results in a complication ratio of 1 complication for every 2.6 bone block distraction subtalar arthrodesis procedures performed for calcaneal malunion. Minor complications accounted for 82 total complications resulting in a minor complication rate of 29.5% and a complication per procedure ratio of 1 for every 3.4 procedures. As for the reported major complications, 24 occurred leading to a major complication rate of 8.6% and a complication per procedure ratio of 1 for every 11.6 procedures. Unfortunately, because of the small number of complications in each subgroup, we were unable to determine an odds ratio. Accordingly, we combined the major and minor soft tissue complications into one category and major and minor bone complications into another. Further, because the incidence of complications is generally accepted to be associated with experience in performing a specific surgical approach, we sought to determine if the number of procedures performed by the investigators had any correlation with soft tissue and/or bone complications. To define proficiency, we arbitrarily selected more than 15 as being an experienced surgeon group and ≤15 procedures being an inexperienced surgeon group. **Tables 1** and **2** represent soft tissue and bone complications, respectively, for comparison of the number of procedures and publication year. The Fisher exact test was performed to determine P values of .0079 and .00047, respectively. Setting our P values for significance at less than 0.05 indicates both **Tables 1** and **2** are statistically significant for our variables. Focusing on the complications data set separated by number of procedures, the incidence of all soft tissue–related complications was 6.3 times higher in those studies with ≤15 procedures included (see **Table 1**). The incidence of all bone-related complications was 2.4 times higher in those studies with ≤15 procedures included (see **Table 2**).

Type of graft used for the bone block arthrodesis was extrapolated. A total of 222 (80%) of the bone blocks were autografts harvested from the patient at time of surgery. Of these autografts, 176 were from the iliac crest, 14 from the resected lateral

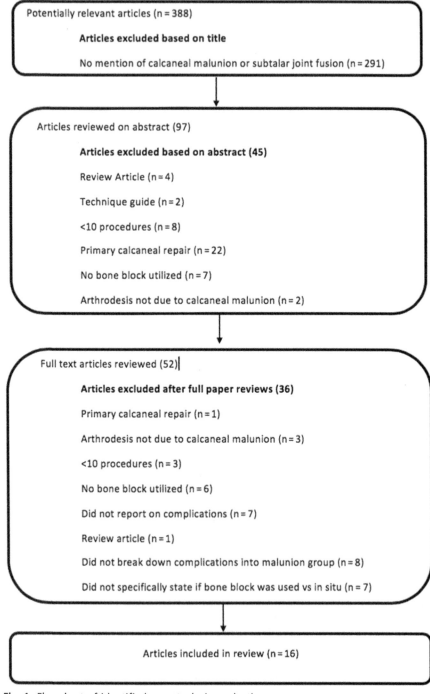

Fig. 1. Flowchart of identified reports during selection process.

Table 3
Specific information included systematic review and meta-analysis

Investigator(s), y (LOE[a])	Mean Age	Procedures	Follow-up, mo	Graft Type	Union	Complications S: Soft Tissue B: Bone	Incisional Approach	Hardware Removal at Time of Surgery	Coleman Methodology Score
Carr et al,[9] 1988 (IV)	NR	11	22	A-ICBG[b]	90.91%	Minor: Soft tissue-7 Bone-5 Major: Soft tissue-0 Bone-3	Posterior-lateral	NR[c]	44
Myerson & Quill,[15] 1993 (IV)	37	14	32	A-ICBG	92.86%	Minor: Soft tissue- 2 Bone-7 Major: Soft tissue-0 Bone- 2	Lateral	NR	44
Amendola & Lammens,[16] 1996 (IV)	43	15	NR	A-ICBG	100%	Minor: Soft tissue-2 Bone-1 Major: Soft tissue-0 Bone-1	Lateral	NR	53
Bednarz et al,[17] 1997 (IV)	44	19	33	A-ICBG	89.47%	Minor: Soft tissue-1 Bone-0 Major: Soft tissue-0 Bone- 5	Posterior-lateral	NR	63
Burton et al,[18] 1998 (IV)	56	13	45	A-ICBG	100%	Minor: Soft tissue-2 Bone-1 Major: Soft tissue-0 Bone-0	Lateral	NR	49
Chen et al,[19] 1998 (IV)	36	32	64	A-ICBG	96.88%	Minor: Soft tissue-2 Bone- 7 Major: Soft tissue-1 Bone- 1	Lateral	NR	54
Marti et al,[20] 1999 (IV)	48	23	108	A-ICBG	95.65%	Minor: Soft tissue-1 Bone-0 Major: Soft tissue-1 Bone-1	Posterior-lateral	NR	54

(continued on next page)

Table 3
(continued)

Investigator(s), y (LOE^a)	Mean Age	Procedures	Follow-up, mo	Graft Type	Union	Complications S: Soft Tissue B: Bone	Incisional Approach	Hardware Removal at Time of Surgery	Coleman Methodology Score
Baravarian[12] 2004 (IV)	NR	12	Minimum of 2 mo	A-ICBG-4 AL^d-8	100%	Minor: Soft tissue-0 Bone-0 Major: Soft tissue-0 Bone-1	Posterior-lateral Lateral when previous ORIF	7	51
Rammelt & Zwipp,[3] 2004 (III)	38.5	31	33	A-ICBG	100%	Minor: Soft tissue-2 Bone-1 Major: Soft tissue-0 Bone-1	Posterior-lateral	11	79
Pollard & Schuberth,[21] 2008 (IV)	46.7	13	27.3	A-ICBG - 8 A-CBG^e-3 AL-ICBG^f -2	100%	Minor: Soft tissue-6 Bone-4 Major: Soft tissue-0 Bone-0	Posterior-lateral	Yes, but NR	49
Lee & Tallerico,[22] 2010 (IV)	47.5	13	20.6	AL	92.31%	Minor: Soft tissue-5 Bone-5 Major: Soft tissue-1 Bone-1	Posterior-lateral	3	43
Wu et al,[23] 2010 (IV)	41	32	34	A^g	100%	Minor: Soft tissue- 1 Bone-0 Major: Soft tissue-0 Bone-0	Lateral	NR	46
Al-Ashhab,[24] 2012 (IV)	28.7	11	13.5	A-CBG	100%	Minor: Soft tissue-2 Bone-0 Major: Soft tissue-3 Bone- 0	Lateral	NR	56
Chiang et al,[25] 2013 (IV)	51	15	36	AL-FHBG^h	100%	Minor: Soft tissue-1 Bone-1 Major: Soft tissue-1 Bone-1	Posterior-lateral	NR	53

Study				Graft	Fusion	Complications	Approach		
Henning et al,[13] 2015 (IV)	45.7	12	14	A-ICBG-6 X-BBG[i]-6	92%	Minor: Soft tissue-10 Bone-4 Major: Soft tissue-1 Bone-1	Lateral	NR	51
Monaco et al,[26] 2016 (IV)	43.9	12	7.7	AL-FHBG[j]	100%	Minor: Soft tissue-1 Bone-1 Major: Soft tissue-0 Bone-0	Lateral	2	27
Totals	42.6	278	40.3	Autograft: 222 ICBG: 176 CB: 14 NR: 32 Allograft: 50 FHBG:27 NR: 21 ICBG: 2 Xenograft: 6 BBG: 6	95.78%	Minor: Soft tissue-45 Bone-37 Major: Soft tissue-6 Bone-18 Total: 106	Lateral: 148 (9) Posterior-lateral: 130 (8)	23	53.15

Major: complete nerve loss, infection requiring further incision and drainage, nonunion, malunion, osteotomies; Minor: superficial soft tissue infection, temporary paresthesia, exostosis, hardware removal.

Abbreviations: A, autograft; A-CBG, autograft calcaneal bone graft; A-ICBG, autograft iliac crest bone graft; AL, allograft; AL-CBG, allograft calcaneal bone graft; AL-FHBG, allograft femoral head bone graft; AL-ICBG, allograft iliac crest bone graft; NR, not reported; X-BBG, xenograft bovine bone graft.

a Level of evidence.
b Autograft iliac crest bone graft.
c Not reported.
d Allograft.
e Autograft calcaneal bone graft.
f Allograft illiac crest bone graft.
g Autograft.
h Allograft femoral head bone graft.
i Xenograft bovine bone graft.
j Allograft femoral head bone graft.

wall of the calcaneus, and in 32 of the autografts the origin was not reported. Allografts were used for the bone block arthrodesis in 50 (18%) of the procedures, with 27 being femoral head/neck and 2 iliac crest, and in 21 the origin of the allograft was not reported. In the study performed by Henning and colleagues,[13] there were 6 bone blocks that were bovine xenografts. Unfortunately, because of the limited information presented in each publication for type of bone graft used and complications that occurred, we were not able to analyze this further. However, on face value, it appeared that the use of autogenous bone graft as the primary source of bone graft declined after 2004. We surmised that the year of publication could serve as a surrogate marker for source of bone graft and complications. Accordingly, we arbitrarily selected publications before 2005 as reflecting the period of primarily autogenous bone graft utilization and 2005 and later as reflecting the period of less autogenous bone graft utilization. The incidence of all soft tissue–related complications was 1.7 times higher in those studies published in 2005 and later (see **Table 1**). The incidence of all bone-related complications was 1.8 times higher in those studies published before 2005 (see **Table 2**).

Looking deeper into **Tables 1** and **2**, there are further trends we are able to observe. In **Table 1**, analyzing the soft tissue complications, it is interesting to note that of the 7 total complications in the studies with more than 15 procedures, 6 (85.7%) of these occurred before 2005. Although in the publications with ≤15 procedures, of the 44 soft tissue complications, 31 (70.45%) happened after 2005. Similarly, when looking at the bone complications (see **Table 2**), all complications (16) that occurred in studies with more than 15 procedures happened before 2005. Studies with more than 15 procedures yielded 39 total bone complications of which 21 (54%) happened before 2005 and 18 (46%) after 2005. As mentioned previously, P values indicate statistical significance of **Tables 1** and **2**.

The methodological quality of all included studies was rated as fair. All but 1 of the studies that met our inclusion criteria were level IV evidence-based medicine studies according to the American College of Foot and Ankle Surgeons Evidence-Based Medicine Chart (https://www.acfas.org/Education-and-Professional-Development/Annual-Scientific-Conference/Manuscript-Submission/; accessed August 6, 2018) (see **Table 3**). All studies included in our review were published in peer-reviewed journals. The mean weighted Coleman Methodology Score was 53.2 ± 10.8 (27–79) for all 16 studies.[14]

DISCUSSION

DIACF remains a challenging condition to treat, requiring a highly specialized skill set to optimize patient outcomes and limit the potential life-altering complications. Many salvage procedures have been described for the known complications associated with DIACF; however, bone block distraction arthrodesis has been demonstrated to afford restoration of calcaneal height and length, varus correction, and resolution of posttraumatic subtalar joint arthritis.[3,9,12–26] We undertook this systematic review specifically for distraction bone block arthrodesis to address calcaneal malunion following DIACF, as we identified some deficiencies in the prior systematic review on this topic. The systematic review of Schepers[8] included 456 patients from 21 studies and demonstrated a 4% nonunion incidence; however, not all included studies reported on complications. Specifically, at least 2 studies did not specify that the complications listed came from the distraction bone block subtalar joint group. This left a total of 421 patients in whom complications could be accounted for. The most common complication noted was hardware removal in 41 patients. There were 13 instances of malunion with no mention of further treatment. Superficial wounding and neural complications were also reported. Unfortunately, there was no mention or calculation of complication rates per patient or procedure, nor were complications stratified per study. We identified a total of 16 studies involving 278 procedures with a weighted bone union rate of 95.78%. This is similar to the union rate reported by Schepers[8] that was 96% for all studies included and minimally reduced to 95% when studies with fewer than 10 procedures were excluded from his analysis. The incidence of union with distraction bone block arthrodesis seems unexpectedly high when compared with union following primary subtalar arthrodesis regardless of technique being up to 35%.[27] Easley and colleagues[28] reported on 109 subtalar joint arthrodeses performed due to calcaneal malunions, including both bone block distraction and in situ arthrodesis, with an overall union rate of 88%. In a study by Catanzariti and colleagues[29] of primary subtalar joint arthrodesis for multiple etiologies, the nonunion rate was 10%. Ziegler and colleagues[27] determined a 23.8% nonunion rate for primary subtalar joint arthrodesis to treat posttraumatic arthritis that was not different from the 23.6% nonunion rate for those undergoing revision subtalar joint arthrodesis. They determined that the nonunion rate when all risk factors were excluded was still 12% despite no bone block being included. Comparing these nonunion rates with the 4.22% nonunion rate found in our study does raise the question of why is there such a contrast in union rates. It is possible that in revision subtalar joint arthrodesis there is greater attention paid to bone bed preparation to expose bleeding subchondral cancellous substrate. Using a distraction bone block technique may also allow for enhanced intrinsic compression due to the tension placed across the fusion sites from the contracted periarticular soft tissues being acutely stretched. There also may be a greater use of enhanced fixation constructs across the arthrodesis site that were not formally included in the publications. We identified the incidence of all bone-related complications as 2.4 times higher in those studies with ≤15 procedures included. This intuitively makes sense, as the complicated surgical techniques necessary to properly correct a calcaneal malunion requires advanced understanding of the index traumatic injury, the reason for failure, the correction necessary to achieve optimal foot function, determination of the most advantageous bone graft material source, and the steps involved in delivering appropriate fixation. The learning curve would therefore seem highly dependent on surgeon experience with this surgery. Further, we identified the incidence of all bone-related complications as 1.9 times higher in those studies published before 2005, the period of primary autogenous bone graft utilization. Although this seems counterintuitive, it is possible that the means of determining a clinically symptomatic nonunion and therefore threshold for operative intervention to address this has changed during our publication categories. For example, noncontrast computerized tomography scan use was not commonly used during the period of most publications in our group before 2005. Reliance solely on persistent pain, swelling, or radiographic evidence of internal fixation migration or loosening to define symptomatic nonunion may have artificially increased the number of bone-related complications identified. This unfortunately remains a matter for conjecture.

One of the most common major bone-related complications besides nonunion was a varus malunion. Radiographic measurements were not the focus of our present study, although this does warrant discussion. Rammelt and Zwipp[3] reported on radiographic measures before and after bone block distraction arthrodesis for treatment of calcaneal malunion after DIACF. They reported that 6 of the 8 patients with more than 5° preoperative hindfoot varus deformity were corrected to neutral. Similarly, all 3 cases with more than 10° valgus malalignment were corrected to neutral. Although a small sample size, these findings do support the notion that varus malalignment may persist following bone block distraction subtalar joint arthrodesis. Calcaneal height and length are primary concerns to restore, and Rammelt and Zwipp[3] stated in 21 patients there was more than 20% shortening of the calcaneus in comparison with the contralateral side before the revision surgery. They reported that the shortening was fully corrected in only 15 of the 21 patients, again iterating the important point of restoring calcaneal height. It may be possible that part of the learning curve is understanding the need to anticipate this amount of calcaneal shortening that would, in effect, leave a portion of the varus deformity uncorrected.

We identified an inverse correlation between incidence of total soft tissue complications and procedure volume compared with publication date. Specifically, we identified the incidence of all soft tissue–related complications was 6.3 times higher in those studies with ≤15 procedures included and 1.7 times higher in those studies published in 2005 and later. It is intuitive that surgeon experience would have an effect on soft tissue complications because excessive dissection, rough tissue handling, long surgery duration, and prolonged or repeated tourniquet time can predictably lead to greater soft tissue complications. However, the higher incidence of soft tissue complications in more recent publications seems counterintuitive. It is possible that the investigators had a lower threshold for operative intervention for soft tissue wounding/infection or that chronic pain syndromes and nerve-related injuries were more frequently diagnosed after 2005. An area of interest is also the origin of the study, of the 32 soft tissue complications after 2005, 13 complications were reported in the publications originating in the United States, whereas 19 were reported overseas. Medical practice and classification of complications may also play a role in these results. Ultimately, we remain uncertain as to why these trends existed and it is likely that our surrogate marker for bone graft source, year of publication, is at fault.

The Coleman Methodology Score (CMS) was introduced in 2000 as a way to rate studies based on certain biases.[14] The range of possible scores is from zero to 100.[14] The mean weighted CMS for all studies included in our review was 53.2 (see **Table 3**). A score of 100 would indicate lowest level of potential bias, whereas a score of zero indicates a high potential for bias and influence on the data presented.[14] The mid-range CMS identified for the studies included in our review indicate a potential for unresolved bias. However, the included studies are all that is available in the literature worldwide and until higher evidence-based medicine studies are conducted, the potential influence this bias has on outcomes remains unanswered.

Unfortunately, like all systematic reviews, limitations to our work exist. Only studies with ≥10 surgeries were included. This excluded some studies that otherwise would have met our inclusion criteria, rendering that we did not include all available studies. Multiple peer-reviewed studies with larger patient populations were excluded simply due to reporting complications as a whole and for not identifying the indication for the bone block distraction subtalar joint arthrodesis. We had very specific inclusion criteria with the indication for surgery needing to be a calcaneal malunion following DIACF and the procedure had to involve the distraction bone block technique. Although we mention the strict inclusion criteria as a limitation, it did allow us to focus on a specific topic to get the most accurate data. Another limitation would be no exclusion criteria based on duration of follow-up. One article did not record follow-up, but did indicate patients were followed until fusion or nonunion could be determined. Another study recorded only a minimum follow-up of 2 months. The use of only electronic databases also can be seen as a limitation, as it is possible studies not available electronically may have been published and not discovered due to our methods. However, we were able to identify a total of 388 articles, as well as search all available references to identify the 16 studies included in our analysis. Our pooled cohort data revealed a total of 106 complications in the 278 procedures. This amounts to a 38% complication rate for all procedures performed, although an individual patient may have more than 1 complication. Unfortunately, we were unable to determine the true incidence of minor versus major soft tissue and bone complications, and also could not determine the effect of bone graft source on the incidence of complications. However, based on our surrogate measures of procedure number and year of publication, we did identify that the incidence of total bone and soft tissue complications reduces with greater surgeon experience, which is intuitive. We unexpectedly identified a greater incidence of total bone complications in the period of greater autograft use and higher incidence of soft tissue complications in the period of less autograft use. These findings warrant further study. Finally, we used a subjective scoring system to report on bias for our included studies, which may be seen as a limitation, although the CMS is a well-known scoring system to report potential bias that is an important consideration.

In conclusion, we present a systematic review and quantitative synthesis on subtalar joint bone block distraction arthrodesis for calcaneal malunion following DIACF. There were 16 studies included with a total of 278 procedures. The weighted mean union rate of all procedures was 95.78%, much higher than those published for primary subtalar joint arthrodesis, although comparable to the 96% union rate identified in the systematic review by Schepers.[8] Of the 278 procedures included, 106 total complications for an incidence rate of 38% occurred, of which 24 were considered major and 82 minor complications. All studies included except 1 were level IV evidence-based medicine studies. This leaves ample opportunity for more methodologically sound studies to be performed on this topic. All procedures noted were open procedures, leaving data on newer techniques and percutaneous approaches unexplored. Our data also support the difficulty of this procedure even in the skilled hands of experienced surgeons and suggests further emphasis is necessary to evaluate the role of modern techniques involving robust internal fixation, advanced osteobiologic grafting options,[30] and minimal soft tissue dissection while limiting potential for soft tissue–related complications.

ACKNOWLEDGMENTS

The authors thank Luis Rameriez, MS, for his assistance in the statistical analysis of their quantitative synthesis.

REFERENCES

1. Clare MP, Crawford WS. Managing complications of calcaneus fractures. Foot Ankle Clin 2017;22:105–16.
2. O'Connell F, Mital MA, Rowe CR. Evaluation of modern management of fractures of the os calcis. Clin Orthop Relat Res 1972;8:214–23.
3. Rammelt S, Zwipp H. Fractures of the calcaneus: current treatment strategies. Acta Chir Orthop Traumatol Cech 2014;81:177–96.
4. Monaco S, Calderone M, Fleming J. Paradigm shift for the surgical management of calcaneal fractures? Clin Podiatr Med Surg 2018;35:175–82.
5. Sangeorzan BJ, Wagner UA, Harrington RM, et al. Contact characteristics of the subtalar joint: the effect of talar neck misalignment. J Orthop Res 1992;10: 544–51.
6. Stapelton J, Belczyk R, Zgonis T. Surgical treatment of calcaneal fracture malunions and post-traumatic deformities. Clin Podiatr Med Surg 2009;26:79–90.

7. Yu X, Pang QJ, Chen L, et al. Post-operative complications after closed calcaneus fracture treated by open reduction and internal fixation: a review. J Int Med Res 2014;42:17–25.

8. Schepers T. The subtalar distraction bone block arthrodesis following the late complications of calcaneal fractures: a systematic review. Foot (Edinb) 2013; 23:39–44.

9. Carr JB, Hansen ST, Benirschke SK. Subtalar distraction bone block fusion for late complications of os calcis fractures. Foot Ankle 1988;9:81–6.

10. Banerjee R, Saltzman C, Anderson RB, et al. Management of calcaneal malunion. J Am Acad Orthop Surg 2011;19:27–36.

11. Barendregt JJ, Doi SA, Lee YY, et al. Meta-analysis of prevalence. J Epidemiol Community Health 2013;67:974–8.

12. Baravarian B. Block distraction arthrodesis for the treatment of failed calcaneal fractures. Clin Podiatr Med Surg 2004;21:241–50.

13. Henning C, Poglia G, Anderson-Leie M, et al. Comparative study of subtalar arthrodesis after calcaneal fracture malunion with autologous bone graft or freeze-dried xenograft. J Exp Orthop 2015;2:10.

14. Coleman BD, Khan KM, Maffulli N, et al. Studies of surgical outcome after patellar tendinopathy: clinical significance of methodological deficiencies and guidelines for future studies. Scand J Med Sci Sports 2000;10:2–11.

15. Myerson M, Quill GE Jr. Late complications of fractures of the calcaneus. J Bone Joint Surg Am 1993;75:331–41.

16. Amendola A, Lammens P. Subtalar arthrodesis using interposition iliac crest bone graft after calcaneal fracture. Foot Ankle Int 1996;17:608–14.

17. Bednarz PA, Beals TC, Manoli A II. Subtalar distraction bone block fusion: an assessment of outcome. Foot Ankle Int 1997;18:785–91.

18. Burton DC, Olney BW, Horton GA. Late results of subtalar distraction fusion. Foot Ankle Int 1998;19:197–202.

19. Chen YJ, Huang TJ, Hsu KY, et al. Subtalar distractional realignment arthrodesis with wedge bone grafting and lateral decompression for calcaneal malunion. J Trauma 1998;45:729–37.

20. Marti RK, de Heus JA, Roolker W, et al. Subtalar arthrodesis with correction of deformity after fractures of the os calcis. J Bone Joint Surg Br 1999;81:611–6.

21. Pollard JD, Schuberth JM. Posterior bone block distraction arthrodesis of the subtalar joint: a review of 22 cases. J Foot Ankle Surg 2008;47:191–8.

22. Lee MS, Tallerico V. Distraction arthrodesis of the subtalar joint using allogeneic bone graft: a review of 15 cases. J Foot Ankle Surg 2010;49:369–74.

23. Wu Y, Wang Y, Wang JH, et al. Treatment of malunited calcaneus fracture with subtalar distraction bone block fusion. Zhonghua Wai Ke Za Zhi 2010;48:655–7.

24. Al-Ashhab MEA. Treatment for calcaneal malunion. Eur J Orthop Surg Traumatol 2013;23:961–6.

25. Chiang C-C, Tzeng Y-H, Lin C-F, et al. Subtalar distraction arthrodesis using fresh-frozen allogeneic femoral head augmented with local autograft. Foot Ankle Int 2013;34:550–6.

26. Monaco SJ, Brandao RA, Manway JM, et al. Subtalar distraction arthrodesis with fresh frozen femoral neck allograft a retrospective case series. Foot Ankle Spec 2016;9:423–8.

27. Ziegler P, Friederichs J, Hungerer S. Fusion of the subtalar joint for post-traumatic arthrosis: a study of functional outcomes and non-unions. Int Orthop 2017;41: 1387–93.

28. Easley ME, Trnka HJ, Schon LC, et al. Isolated subtalar arthrodesis. J Bone Joint Surg Am 2000;82:613–24.
29. Catanzariti AR, Medicino RW, Saltrick KR, et al. Subtalar joint arthrodesis. J Am Podiatr Med Assoc 2005;95:34–41.
30. Magnus M, Iceman K, Roukis TS. Living cryopreserved bone allograft as an adjunct for hindfoot arthrodesis. Clin Podiatr Med Surg 2018;35:295–310.

Wound Coverage Options for Soft Tissue Defects Following Calcaneal Fracture Management (Operative/Surgical)

Christopher Bibbo, DO, DPM[a,*], Noman Siddiqui, DPM, MHA[b],
Jessica Fink, DPM[c], Jake Powers, DPM[d,e], David A. Ehrlich, MD[f],
Steven J. Kovach, MD[g]

KEYWORDS

- Calcaneus • Fracture • Wounds • Incision • Flaps

KEY POINTS

- Calcaneus fractures are a life-changing event, and the soft tissue injury with attendant healing complications possesses the potential for significant morbidity.
- The management of soft tissue complications with calcaneus fractures follows a progressive stepwise algorithm, from the simplest strategy to the most complex.
- In addition to soft tissue defects, simultaneous bone defects also may require reconstruction; in this instance, the combination of soft tissue and bone flaps may provide a composite tissue to meet the reconstructive requirements.
- Amputation is the final option for injuries that are unable to be reconstructed.
- Following sound orthoplastic principles in the management of soft tissue defects associated with calcaneal fractures is paramount.

Disclosures: No authors have any disclosures and or commercial or financial conflicts of interest.
[a] Foot and Ankle Section, Plastic Reconstructive and Microsurgery, Musculoskeletal Infection Service, Limb Salvage, and Orthopaedic Trauma, Rubin Institute for Advanced Orthopaedics, Sinai Hospital of Baltimore, Baltimore, MD, USA; [b] Diabetic Limb Preservation at Lifebridge Health, Rubin Institute for Advanced Orthopaedics, Sinai Hospital of Baltimore, 2401 West Belvedere Avenue, Baltimore, MD 21215, USA; [c] Rubin Institute for Advanced Orthopaedics, Sinai Hospital of Baltimore, 2401 West Belvedere Avenue, Baltimore, MD 21215, USA; [d] Sinai Hospital of Baltimore, Baltimore, VA, 2401 West Belvedere Avenue, Baltimore, MD 21215, USA; [e] Foot and Ankle Surgery Residency, Baltimore, MD, USA; [f] Reconstructive and Plastic Surgery, Private Practice, 840 Walnut Street, 15th Floor, Philadelphia, PA 19107, USA; [g] Plastic Reconstructive and Orthopaedic Surgery, University of Pennsylvania Health System, Perelman Center for Advanced Medicine, 3400 Civic Center Boulevard, South Pavilion, 1st Floor, Philadelphia, PA 19104, USA
* Corresponding author. 2809 Boston Street, #105, Baltimore, MD 21224.
E-mail address: drchrisbibbo@gmail.com

Clin Podiatr Med Surg 36 (2019) 323–337
https://doi.org/10.1016/j.cpm.2018.10.012
0891-8422/19/© 2018 Elsevier Inc. All rights reserved.

podiatric.theclinics.com

INTRODUCTION

The calcaneus is the most commonly fractured tarsal bone, most commonly occurring in young men ranging in age from 20 to 39 years, with most fractures associated with high-energy mechanisms (ie, falls from a height, motor vehicle crashes).[1] The operative management of this life-changing fracture is in part due to the often hostile, soft tissue envelope surrounding the hindfoot after fracture. Open fractures display a spectrum of injury, most commonly medial, lateral, posterior, and degloving wounds (**Fig. 1**A–C). Blast injuries with calcaneal fractures, such as in industrial and military settings, pose the highest morbidity. Soft tissue injuries associated with calcaneus fractures also may present late, presenting as an unstable soft tissue envelope (**Fig. 2**) that may be painful, prone to repeated breakdown with drainage, and the development of osteomyelitis.

Wound complications related to surgical incisions are also on a spectrum, from the well-known tip necrosis, dehiscence, and the development of a major area wound

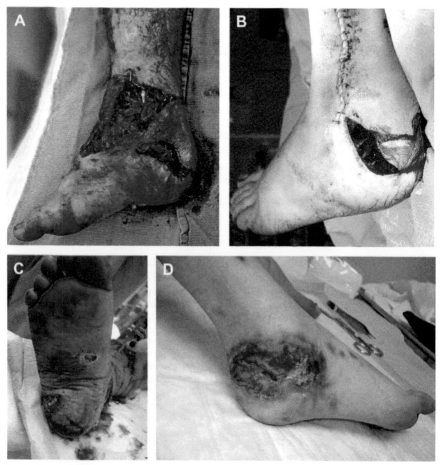

Fig. 1. Photographic examples of open calcaneal wounds: medial (A), posterior (B), and degloving (C) that may result in catastrophic soft tissue loss. Example of a major area wound complication associated with calcaneus fracture (D).

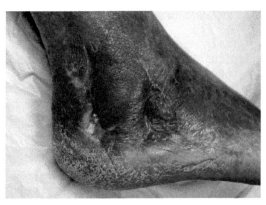

Fig. 2. Late presentation of a painful, unstable soft tissue envelope after calcaneus fracture and surgical management.

complication (**Fig.** 1D). Traditionally, wound healing complications after the lateral extensile approach are reported to range from 5% to 30%.[2–6] Worsening wound complications are associated with open fractures, and severe displacement with contracture of an edematous soft tissue envelope. However, recently the work of Bibbo and colleagues[2] demonstrated that the patency of the lateral calcaneal branch of the peroneal artery, which supplies the lateral calcaneal perferasome, is critical to the prevention of developing wound complications.

Prevention is critical to operative management of calcaneus fracture. This commences with the immediate preoperative period. Edema is a common and well-respected condition that is associated with many fractures, particularly calcaneal fractures. The inflammatory milieu with a state of capillary leak of the injured, edematous soft tissue does not exhibit the appropriate healing as does tissue in the normal physiologic state. Thus, resolution of edema before placing incisions is critical. Regardless of passing trends, edema and fracture blisters need to be well managed following injury, before any surgical intervention. Edema can compromise the cutaneous perforators, resulting in soft tissue necrosis. Typically, surgery is delayed for 7 to 10 days following injury when soft tissue swelling has subsided. This can be tested clinically as the "wrinkle sign" in which the Langerhans lines are visible, indicating swelling has subsided enough to proceed with open reduction.[6] Immediate and acute surgery (2 to 4 days) with the lateral extensile approach imparts the risk for minor and major wound healing complications. Second, preventing a contracted soft tissue envelope is important. The restoration of calcaneal height and elimination of displaced fracture fragments "tenting the skin" in severely depressed/displaced calcaneal fractures is best suited by temporary restoration of height, such as by the use of temporary Steinman pins through the calcaneal tuber-body, the use of small external fixators, and at times, fine wire circular fixation. Third, in the setting of open fractures, urgent and meticulous management of the soft tissue of the open fractures is paramount for the prevention of wound healing complication. Moreover, when calcaneal fractures are at risk for infection, at the time of surgery, it has been demonstrated that the use of human demineralized bone matrix, in combination with antibiotics, may provide an excellent augment to bone healing and prevention of infection after open reduction and internal fixation (ORIF) of calcaneal fractures, without adverse effects.[7]

The prevention of wound healing complication is, however, most likely impacted the greatest by adequacy of blood flow to the lateral calcaneal soft tissue envelope; thus,

Doppler examination of the lateral calcaneal artery is mandatory before incision on the lateral calcaneus.[2]

The significance of incision planning is an important feature in the development of wound healing complications along the lateral wall of the calcaneus. The lateral extensile approach, first described by LeTournel, and later popularized by Benirschke and Sangeorzan, is one of the most commonly used incisions.[8] This L-shaped incision is created with the perpendicular arm just anterior to the Achilles tendon and the horizontal arm following the glabrous junction, between the lateral and plantar heel. The key to the success of this incision is, again, perfusion to the lateral calcaneal skin supplied by the lateral calcaneal artery, a branch from the peroneal artery. The peroneal artery travels alongside the fibula in the deep compartment, the terminal branch being the lateral calcaneal artery. The lateral calcaneal artery exits the deep crural fascia at a mean of 3.8 cm above the midpoint of a line that extends from the tip of the lateral malleolus, to the calcaneal insertion of Achilles tendon, and mean of 2.5 cm posterior to lateral malleolus. At this intersection zone, the mean vessel diameter is approximately 1.75 mm. At the level of the ankle, the superficial course of the peroneal/lateral calcaneal artery junction is maximally at risk in the lower leg.[9] However, the artery is at constant risk from both trauma and incisions within its entire lateral course. Thus, interruption of the lateral calcaneal artery places most of the lateral perferasome over the calcaneus in jeopardy.[2] Ultimately, the lateral calcaneal branch gives 4 to 5 perforators to the soft tissue envelope before terminating.[6] Small lateral terminal branches for the tibialis anterior artery ramify with the lateral calcaneal artery over the sinus tarsi and at the level of the subtalar joint. Thus, the lateral extensile approach is placed between the perferasomes of the lateral calcaneal artery and the lateral terminal branches of the plantar lateral artery, delineated at the lateral skin glabrous junction; the entire soft tissue flap is elevated on essentially the lateral calcaneal branch of the peroneal artery.[2,10] Patency of the lateral calcaneal artery is paramount, and easily performed with a Doppler probe.

Recently, with the introduction of a proprietary periarticular buttress plate, variations of the McReynold approach, based just below the level of the subtalar joint, has been repopularized. The authors advise caution in this zone: in the face of trauma, it is a poor location for the creation of an extensile approach, as it reached the proximal limits of the lateral perferasome and is supplied by a lesser perfusion of the terminal branches of the anterior tibial artery.

WOUNDS AND COVERAGE

All wounds related to calcaneal fractures have the potential for significant morbidity. The goal of the management of wounds is the restoration of the composite layers of the soft tissue envelope. The reconstruction of any soft tissue defect entails abiding by the concept of the "reconstructive ladder," whereas the simplest care strategy is attempted first, followed by sequential implementation of more complex techniques to achieve wound coverage. For example, local wound care would be followed by negative-pressure dressings; subsequent option may include reduction osteoplasty, local flap coverage, and microvascular free tissue transfer. With time and experience gained, the surgeon will recognize if simpler measure needs to be bypassed, and more complex procedures initial at the onset of operative care ("reconstructive elevator"). Adjunctive measures include hyperbaric oxygen treatment, primary negative-pressure dressing, and along the incision, locally delivered growth factors and antibiotics (only if infection is present). Edema control is a constant measure at all times in the perioperative period.

Local Wound Care

Local tissue rearrangement with delayed primary closure is the choice for smaller wounds associated with a supple soft tissue envelope (**Fig. 3**). The use of local wound care measures is indicated as a first-line measure in all wounds that cannot be closed in a delayed primary fashion. The basic premise of local care is to promote an environment for healing (reduction of bacterial colonization, treatment of infection, changing a chronic milieu to one of an acute wound, where healing is better supported).[11] Excess moisture is balanced toward a normal status and vice versa. It is paramount that no matter the wound size, adequate debridement to relatively healthy tissue be performed as often as needed.

Normal sterile saline wet-to-damp 3 or 4 times per day is the starting point; this is especially appropriate for small wounds (incision gaping, tip necrosis, small full-thickness wounds), even large wounds require basic wound care measures while being prepared for operative procedures. Antibiotic ointments and nonadherent dressings have a role in very simple wounds. For larger wounds, silver sulfadiazine 1% (Pfizer, Inc., New York, NY) is a good alternative to maintain proper wound hydration with prophylactic antimicrobial action. Silver dressings for drier wounds, as well as collagenases and alginates for hyperhidrotic fibrous wounds; do have roles in treatment for soft tissue defects.

Negative-Pressure Wound Dressings

The use of negative-pressure wound dressings (NPWDs) is not only an adjunct, but may be indicated as a primary modality for wounds. In wounds that maintain a deep layer of healthy vascularized tissue, a base of granulation may be achieved, allowing wounds to heal secondarily,[12] or can be covered with a skin graft. The use of neo-dermal substrates is helpful in clean wounds, but contraindicated in heavily colonized or infected wounds.

In the setting of staged reconstructions, NPWD is an alternative to promote healing by reducing the volume of inflammatory mediator-laden fluids and via the technique of intermittent delivery of antimicrobial fluids and surfactant agents. The lead author's protocol for grossly contaminated/infected wounds (in conjunction with debridements) is an intermittent instillation of one-quarter to one-half strength sodium hypochlorite solution (Dakin solution; Century Pharmaceuticals, Inc., Indianapolis, IN) for 24 to 48 hours, followed by normal saline, a surfactant, for 24 hours, then standard NPWD techniques. Dilute acetic acid (*Pseudomonas* species infections) or customized

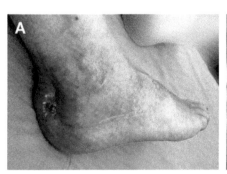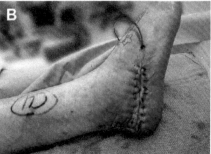

Fig. 3. Small defect related to a calcaneus fracture (*A*). Local tissue rearrangement and delayed primary (*B*).

antibiotic solutions also may be used, most often secondarily or when indicated, as a primary measure. Culture-specific antibiotics and local antibiotic delivery devices are performed in persistent infections, being debrided as often as indicated.

Reduction Osteoplasty

The volumetric reduction of the bone to achieve wound closure was first described by Bibbo in 2005.[3,13] Using this concept, in the setting of wound dehiscence of the lateral extensile approach, a near match of either coronal or frontal plane bone resection can result in a corresponding width of a wound, achieving primary wound closure. The limitation of this technique is related to maintaining enough bone length to not impair functional capacity of the ankle and subtalar joints.

FLAPS: DEFINITIONS AND GENERAL CONSIDERATIONS

Flaps represent the use of tissue composites transferred to a wound defect, either from a local or regional source, in which the vascular corridor to the flap (source pedicle vessels and arterioles/capillaries) is maintained. Free tissue transfers are tissue composites that require the interruption of a source vessel and the reestablishment of flow via microvascular anastomosis with a recipient vessel.

The cardinal rules of all flap surgery are to use tissue that resides a relative distance from the zone of injury (fracture and incision) and infection must be well controlled. Uncontrolled or poorly treated infections will result in flap failure. Next, the use of similar tissue to replace tissue is desired (Gilles principle). Flap durability from exposure to pressure and shearing forces is mandatory.

Local Flaps

A fairly large number of local flaps exist for the coverage of wounds associated with the operative management of calcaneal wounds, both from incisions or open wounds.

The lateral calcaneal artery flap (LCA flap) was first described in 1981.[14] This is an axial pattern flap that includes the lateral calcaneal artery, small distal branches of the lesser saphenous vein, and the sural nerve. The LCA flap has been believed to be a viable option even in severely atherosclerotic patients, as the peroneal artery and its terminal branches are least likely to be affected by occlusion.[15] However, the authors believe this is not applicable in trauma cases in which vessel thrombosis is a real threat. The reported advantages of the LCA flap are that it will accommodate coverage of small to moderate-sized wounds, ease of elevation, the relative thinness of the flap, and the minimal donor site morbidity, as it does not sacrifice a major vessel to the foot. The primary disadvantage of the LCA flap is that it is derived from local tissue in close proximity and within the original zone of injury. In addition, adjacent soft tissue is lost by the design of the flap. Venous congestion and sensory disruptions also may occur.[15] The authors consider the LCA flap, with the exception of chronic small wounds, to be a poor flap selection.

The reverse sural flap (Rev Sural) is an option for coverage of the lateral and posterior heel; it is a lesser choice for the plantar heel due to the weight-bearing pressure plantar aspect of the heel. The blood supply to this flap is provided by perforating branches of the peroneal artery. Advantages of the Rev Sural flap include it may be appropriately thin, and may be harvested as a fasciocutaneous or adipofascial flap (in obese patients). In addition, the Rev Sural flap may be designed to accommodate narrow (**Fig. 4**A) or wide (**Fig. 4**B) soft tissue defects. In pediatric patients (see **Fig. 4**B), the Rev Sural is also a reliable flap as a stand-alone or an adjunct flap,[16] and as the

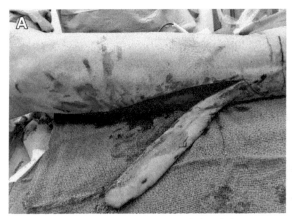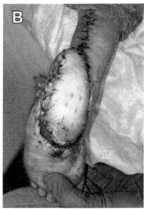

Fig. 4. The reverse sural flap designed thin (A). Reverse sural flap designed wide, in this instance used in a pediatric calcaneus injury (B).

child grows, donor site morbidity is limited (see **Fig. 4**B). This flap, although often reliable, may require delay technique in the multimorbid patient, as complication rates in multimorbid patients exceed 50%.[17] The most common complication encountered with the Rev Sural type of flap is venous congestion, that may result in partial- or full-thickness flap necrosis. Therapies for venous congestion include exteriorization of the short saphenous vein to elute blood and leech therapy; both are continued until cyanosis ceases. Leech therapy is associated with postoperative anemia, often requiring transfusion, as the leech hirudin anticoagulant acts systemically. Leech therapy has the potential for the transmission of drug-resistant organisms,[18] necessitating broad-spectrum antibiotics for at least 2 weeks after leech therapy is discontinued. Partial-thickness flap necrosis may be salvaged by tangential debridement, often with the finding of a viable fascial layer, that can be managed with NPWD to achieve a granulation bed. As long as all exposed bone and/or hardware is covered with the viable portion of the flap; conservative modalities, such as NPWD or routine dressing care, can be instituted for continued healing without any further surgical intervention. The donor site is easily managed with small flaps, but larger flaps (>7 cm wide) will require skin grafting.

The plantar medial artery (PMA) flap is extremely useful for coverage of plantar heel flaps (**Fig. 5**A) that can be seen in very high energy injuries, resulting in plantar blowout of the soft tissue as the calcaneus is nearly extruded from the foot. The PMA flap is also for late reconstruction of unstable plantar calcaneal wounds (**Fig. 5**B). The benefits of this flap include a near identical tissue composite of the plantar heel, a near uniform presence of its pedicle from the PMA, a location away from the zone of injury, and a donor site that is easily managed.

Propeller flaps, generally fasciocutaneous flaps, are designed in the shape of a large ellipse, and are rotated about the anterior leg perforator axis between the fibula and tibia. The design is such that the arc of rotation is similar to motion of a propeller about its axle. The anterolateral propeller flap may have the reach to cover calcaneal wounds alone or in conjunction with the reverse peroneus brevis muscle flap (**Fig. 6**). With near uniformity, the donor site cannot be primarily closed and a skin graft is required. As in all adipofascial flaps, when the fat layer is robust and thick, in-setting of the flap will become a significant issue over the calcaneus, an area that typically has a thin-layered soft tissue envelope.

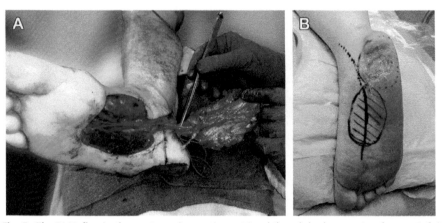

Fig. 5. The PMA flap in the acute perioperative setting (A) and the late setting for a painful unstable plantar heal wound (B).

The lateral supramalleolar flap is a variation of the propeller flap, with the exception that it captures fewer perforators and is based on the perforating peroneal artery, a communicating conduit between the peroneal and anterior tibial arteries. It may also be distally based on the artery of the sinus tarsi, but in the setting of calcaneal fracture, raising a distally based lateral supramalleolar flap is not advised. The donor site morbidity is significant due to its harvest being over the fibula. It is not a desirable flap for wound coverage.

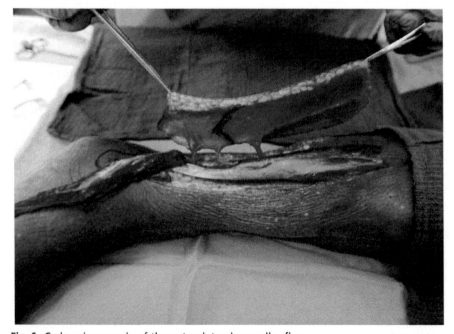

Fig. 6. Cadaveric example of the anterolateral propeller flap.

The intrinsic pedal muscles may be used for reconstruction of calcaneal defects. The most useful intrinsic pedal muscle flaps for calcaneal fractures, soft tissue and bone defects, include the abductor hallucis muscle (ABH) flap and the abductor digiti minimi (quinti) muscle (AbdQ) flap.

The ABH flap is useful for medial calcaneal wounds when raised as a proximally based flap. Medial calcaneal wounds are most commonly from open fractures, and to a lesser degree, from ancillary incisions to assist with reduction and fixation of incarcerated or severely displaced medial fracture fragments. Possessing a type 2 blood supply, an ABH flap may be elevated proximally or distally. The arc of rotation and reach can be increased by detaching it from its origin on the calcaneus. The donor site is easily closed primarily with low donor site morbidity (**Fig. 7**). The ABH flap can be used in conjunction with a PMA advancement/transposition flap for deep plantar defects: the ABH flap fills the deep void, whereas the PMA flap resurfaces the heel pad. Disadvantages of the ABH flap are the variable patient-to-patient size of the muscle and the potential to lie in the zone of injury.

The AbdQ muscle receives its blood supply from the lateral plantar artery, with a proximal perforator and a smaller distal perforator (type 2 blood supply). The AbdQ is a small muscle (**Fig. 8**), extending from the lateral plantar calcaneal tubercle to the lateral base of the fifth digit proximal phalanx, the bulk of the muscle belly is

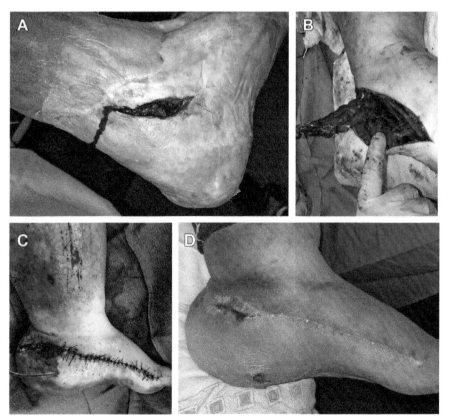

Fig. 7. The ABH flap filling a medial calcaneal bone and soft tissue defect: wound (*A*), flap elevation (*B*), flap inset (*C*), healed (*D*).

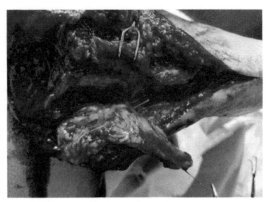

Fig. 8. The abductor digiti minimi (quinti) muscle flap has a limited arc of rotation and size; however, it is useful for wounds along the glabrous junction. (*Courtesy of* Suhail Masedah, DPM, Cincinnati, OH.)

located proximally; thus, its usefulness is limited to small defects along and just proximal to the glabrous skin junction. Advantages include ease of harvest along the glabrous junction, and it is considered a functionally expendable muscle. However, loss of the AbdQ muscle may result in lack of plantar lateral padding, which may result in discomfort; this may be remedied by a soft insert.

Large, deep calcaneal wounds, and those complicated by osteomyelitis, require a larger, more robust muscle flap. The distally based (reverse) peroneus brevis (Rev PB) muscle flap (**Fig. 9** A–C) is a reliable and safe option even in complex cases,[19] offering a way to provide durable and effective coverage while filling anatomic dead space and supplying vascularity. The peroneus brevis muscle has a type 2 blood supply pattern. On average, there are 3 to 6 pedicles supplied by the anterior tibial vessels anteriorly and proximally and the peroneal vessel posteriorly and distally. The average length of the flap is 21 cm in length by 3 cm in width, making it a great option for the large lateral heel defects.[19,20] Advantages include ease of elevation, low donor site morbidity, reliability, reduction of anatomic dead space, and when the peroneus longus and brevis tendons are tenodesed distally, there is minimal biomechanical dysfunction during gait.

Free Tissue Transfers

Simply referred to as a free flap, the hallmark of these flaps is that the blood supply (arterial and venous) of the flap is divided and reestablished by microvascular

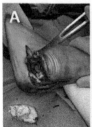
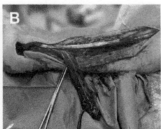
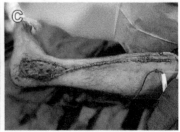

Fig. 9. Large lateral calcaneal soft tissue and bone defect (*A*). Harvest of the reverse peroneus brevis flap (*B*). Flap is inset and skin graft applied (*C*).

anastomosis to recipient vessels in proximity to the defect area. These flaps are tech-nically difficult, require specialized microsurgical training, and are best performed in patients who are able to withstand prolonged general anesthesia. The advantage of free flaps is that all tissue or partial tissue composites are supplied (single tissues/combinations of skin, muscle, and bone), there is a robust bed of vascularized tissue offered, the flaps are generally durable, and there are several options for thin flaps that match the tissue about the lateral calcaneus. A practical disadvantage for free flaps is that the traumatized lower extremity remains the most challenging region for which to be successful.

Indications for free flaps include large soft tissue defects that prohibit the relative limited amount of tissue a local flap (rotation or pedicled) will provide. Criteria for free flaps proposed by Cavadas and Landin[4] include a deficit being larger than 5 cm (infected or not), an infected defect with anatomically reconstructed bone less than 1 month old, noninfected intermediate size (1.5 to 5.0 cm) with distal extension in which the sural flap may not reach, and finally in a failed sural flap. The authors believe that these are simply guidelines, as the need and selection of free flaps has evolved on many levels. However, the failure of local flaps, and the need for vascular-ized bone for calcaneal reconstruction are uniform indications for free flaps.

Preoperative arteriogram with distal run-off to ensure intact free flap vasculature is often performed. Most arterial anastomoses are with the anterior tibial vascular sys-tem, followed by the peroneal and posterior tibial vessel system. Microvascular arterial anastomoses are typically end-to-side, whereas venous anastomosis is performed end-to-end. In skilled, experienced hands, the results of free flap reconstruction in the lower extremity are good, with a reported success rate as high as 95%.[21]

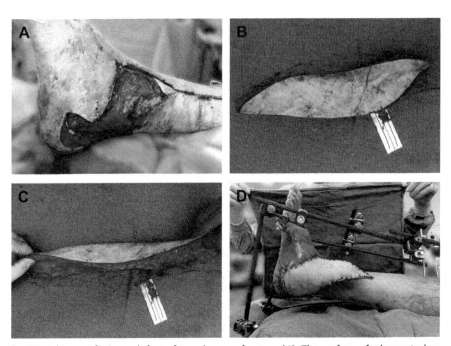

Fig. 10. A large soft tissue defect after calcaneus fracture (*A*). The surface of a harvested an-terolateral thigh free flap (*B*) and profile (*C*) demonstrating a supple, thin flap. The flap inset after microvascular anastomosis (*D*).

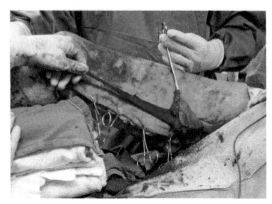

Fig. 11. Harvest of gracilis muscle for use as a free flap.

However, this success rate was a mixed cohort; trauma cases are prone to have greater complications.

Free flaps that may be considered for the calcaneus include the anterolateral thigh (ALT), radial forearm (Rad forearm), gracilis, latissimus dorsi (Latiss D), vertical rectus abdominis (VRAM), and the vastus lateralis (Vastus lat). Among these, the Rad forearm and "thin" ALT free flaps best match the thinner soft tissue envelope of the heel.

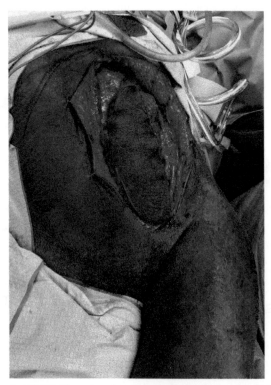

Fig. 12. Elevation of a VRAM. The advantage of the VRAM is a long pedicle with a generous vessel diameter for microvascular anastomosis. Loss of donor site function is offset by the external and internal oblique muscles.

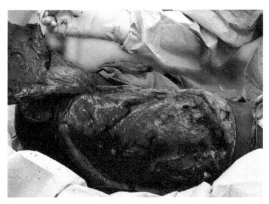

Fig. 13. Elevation of a myocutaneous latissimus dorsi free flap. The advantage of this flap is size, pedicle length, and diameter, and little functional loss.

However, in the authors' opinion, the Rad forearm free flap is quite often inadequate, as typically soft tissue defects over calcaneal implants require a thicker composite of tissues. Thus, the workhorse free flaps for traumatic calcaneal wounds are the ALT (**Fig. 10**), gracilis (**Fig. 11**), and VRAM (**Fig. 12**). Because of its large size, the Latiss D flap is of best use in massive defects of the calcaneus and hindfoot (**Fig. 13**). With the exception of the ALT free flap, the other workhorse free flaps may be taken with skin or muscle only. When vascularized bone is needed, the free fibula is applicable, which may be raised with muscle and/or a skin paddle (**Fig. 14**). An alternative to the free fibula is the iliac crest free flap (**Fig. 15**).

AMPUTATION

Failure of all index and repeat management strategies may indicate amputation. Primary amputation is best decided in the hands of the most experienced surgeons. Regardless of the timing, in many settings, amputation may not be considered a failure, but rather an experienced management decision. In conjunction, the patient's desires for salvage or amputation must be intimately considered and honored. Quite often patients "know their body" better than anyone and have mature insight into their decisions.

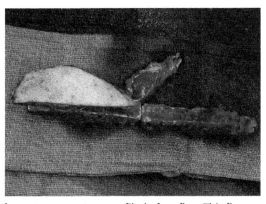

Fig. 14. Example of an osteomyocutaneous fibula free flap. This flap may be used for early or late reconstruction of both soft tissue and bony defects of the calcaneus.

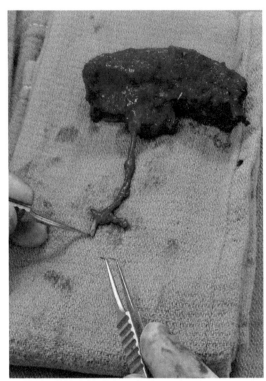

Fig. 15. Free iliac crest bone graft. Although not commonly used, this free flap may be taken with skin for when soft tissue and bone reconstruction are required. The major disadvantages include a short pedicle and pain at the donor site.

SUMMARY

Calcaneus fractures are a life-changing event. Soft tissue injury and the attendant healing complications possess the potential for significant morbidity. This holds true as well for incisions placed for the operative management of calcaneus fractures. The management of soft tissue complications with calcaneus fractures follows a progressive stepwise algorithm, from the simplest strategy to the most complex. In addition to soft tissue defects, simultaneous bone defects may also require reconstruction; in this instance, the combination of soft tissue and bone flaps may provide a composite tissue to meet the reconstructive requirements. Amputation is the final option for injuries that are unable to be reconstructed. Following sound orthoplastic principles in the management of soft tissue defects associated with calcaneal fractures is paramount.

REFERENCES

1. Bohls DD, Ondeck NT, Samuel AM, et al. Demographics, mechanisms of injury, and concurrent injuries associated with calcaneus fractures: a study of 14,516 patients in the American College of Surgeons National Trauma Data Bank. Foot Ankle Spec 2017;10:402–10.
2. Bibbo C, Ehrlich DA, Nyugen HL, et al. Low wound complication rates for the lateral extensile approach for calcaneal ORIF when the lateral calcaneal artery is patent. Foot Ankle Int 2014;35:650–6.

3. Bibbo C. Calcaneal osteotomy for closure of non-healing wounds after ORIF of the calcaneus. Tech Foot Ankle Surg 2005;4:230–4.
4. Cavadas PC, Landin L. Management of soft-tissue complications of the lateral approach for calcaneal fractures. Plast Reconstr Surg 2007;120:459–66.
5. Carow JB, Carow J, Gueorguiev B, et al. Soft tissue micro-circulation in the healthy hindfoot: a cross-sectional study with focus on lateral surgical approaches to the calcaneus. Int Orthop 2018. Available at: https://doi.org/10.1007/s00264-018-4031-7. Accessed September 1, 2018.
6. Attinger C, Cooper P. Soft tissue reconstruction for calcaneal fractures or osteomyelitis. Orthop Clin North Am 2001;32:135–70.
7. Bibbo C, Patel DV. The influence of demineralized bone matrix-calcium sulfate with vancomycin on calcaneus fracture healing and infection rates: a prospective study. Foot Ankle Int 2006;27:487–93.
8. Benirschke SK, Sangeorzan BJ. Extensive intraarticular fractures of the foot. Surgical management of calcaneal fractures. Clin Orthop Relat Res 1993;292:128–34.
9. Elsaidy MA, El-Shaify K. The lateral calcaneal artery: anatomic basis for planning safe surgical approaches. Clin Anat 2009;22:834–9.
10. Borrelli J Jr, Lashgari C. Vascularity of the lateral calcaneal flap: a cadaveric injection study. J Orthop Trauma 1999;13:73–7.
11. Guo S, Dipietro LA. Factors affecting wound healing. J Dent Res 2010;89:219–29.
12. Morykwas MJ, Argenta LC, Shelton-Brown EL, et al. Vacuum-assisted closure: a new method for wound control and treatment: animal studies and basic foundation. Ann Plast Surg 1997;38:553–62.
13. Bibbo C, Stough J. Reduction calcaneoplasty and local muscle rotation flap as a salvage option for calcaneal osteomyelitis with soft tissue defect. J Foot Ankle Surg 2012;51:375–8.
14. Grabb WC, Argenta LC. The lateral calcaneal artery skin flap (the lateral calcaneal artery, lesser saphenous vein and sural nerve skin flap). Plast Reconstr Surg 1981;68:723–30.
15. Burusapat C, Tanthanatip P, Kuhaphensaeng P, et al. Lateral calcaneal artery flaps in atherosclerosis: cadaveric study, vascular assessment and clinical applications. Plast Reconstr Surg Glob Open 2015;3:e517.
16. Bibbo C, Ehrlich DA, Kovach SJ. Pediatric lateral ankle physeal reconstruction by free microvascular transfer of the proximal fibular physis. J Foot Ankle Surg 2015;54:994–1000.
17. Parrett BM, Pribaz JJ, Matros E, et al. Risk analysis for the reverse sural fasciocutaneous flap in distal leg reconstruction. Plast Reconstr Surg 2009;123:1499–504.
18. Bibbo C, Fritsche T, Stemper M, et al. Flap infection associated with medicinal leeches in reconstructive surgery: two new drug-resistant organisms. J Reconstr Microsurg 2013;29:457–60.
19. Rodriguez Collazo ER, Bibbo C, Mechell RJ, et al. The reverse peroneus brevis muscle flap for ankle wound coverage. J Foot Ankle Surg 2013;52:543–6.
20. Masadeh S, Bibbo C. Distally based peroneus brevis flap: a reliable and versatile flap to cover the lateral foot and ankle. Curr Orthop Pract 2016;27:499–507.
21. Attinger CE, Ducic I, Cooper P, et al. The role of intrinsic muscle flaps of the foot for bone coverage in foot and ankle defects in diabetic and nondiabetic patients. Plast Reconstr Surg 2002;110:1047–54.

Salvaging the Unsalvageable Severe Malunion Deformity After Displaced Intra-Articular Calcaneal Fractures
What Options Exist?

Kelli L. Iceman, DPM[a], Mark K. Magnus, DPM[a],
Thomas S. Roukis, DPM, PhD[b],*

KEYWORDS

- Calcanectomy • Calcaneal transplantation • Calcaneal allograft
- Vascularized autograft • Calcaneal prosthesis

KEY POINTS

- Calcaneal malunions are devastating injuries resulting in significant patient morbidity, including periarticular degenerative joint changes, impingement symptoms, gait alterations, and chronic pain.
- Surgical reconstruction is a massive undertaking; the goals are to re-establish the calcaneal height, restore the talocalcaneal relationship, and create a stable, plantigrade foot.
- For treatment of severe calcaneal malunion deformities, potential options include calcanectomy, calcaneal allograft transplantation, vascularized autografts, and calcaneal prosthesis.

INTRODUCTION

Displaced intra-articular calcaneal fractures (DIACFs) continue to be one of the most complex injuries to manage in the lower extremity. Historically, delayed treatment was once preferred due to difficulties associated with acute surgical management and adverse postoperative complications.[1] The significant morbidity, however, associated with conservative treatment of DIACFs has led to favoring more aggressive

Disclosure: Consultant for DePuy Synthes, FH ORTHO, Integra, and Novastep. Royalties received from CrossRoads Extremity, Novastep, and Stryker Orthopaedics.
[a] Gundersen Medical Foundation, Mail Stop CO3-006A, 1900 South Avenue, La Crosse, WI 54601, USA; [b] Orthopaedic Center, Gundersen Health System, Mail Stop CO2-006, 1900 South Avenue, La Crosse, WI 54601, USA
* Corresponding author.
E-mail address: tsroukis@gundersenhealth.org

Clin Podiatr Med Surg 36 (2019) 339–347
https://doi.org/10.1016/j.cpm.2018.10.013
0891-8422/19/© 2018 Elsevier Inc. All rights reserved.

podiatric.theclinics.com

management.[1] Although surgical intervention has become the new standard of treatment, some injuries are so severe that they prohibit primary surgical repair. A fraction of these injuries requiring initial conservative cares may develop into a calcaneal malunion. If the malunion is not addressed in a timely fashion, these displaced fractures often result in debilitating hindfoot and ankle deformities.[2]

CALCANEAL MALUNION OVERVIEW
Anatomy of a Malunion

A drastic change in calcaneal morphology is appreciated in patients with untreated DIACFs. The distorted anatomy causes alterations in the hindfoot and ankle biomechanics, which may lead to a variety of clinical presentations. To appreciate the complex pathoanatomy of a calcaneal malunion, the initial injury and its fracture pattern must be well understood.

Primary fracture

During talar impaction, the lateral process of the talus wedges into the calcaneus (commonly at the angle of Gissane).[3] The resultant fracture is called the primary fracture, which separates the calcaneus into its 2 main fragments: the posterolateral fragment (containing the body and tuberosity) and the superomedial fragment (containing the sustentaculum tali).[3] As a result, the tuberosity fragment translates laterally and superiorly in relation to the sustentaculum fragment. The Böhler angle effectively decreases, thereby causing a decrease in the calcaneal height and an increase in calcaneal width.[1] Displacement of the tuberosity typically results in a varus hindfoot, although a valgus deformity may also occur.[1]

Secondary fractures

As the impaction of the talus continues into the calcaneus, the force dissipates along the length of the calcaneus causing secondary fractures. These fracture lines may produce either a tongue-type fracture pattern, where the fracture extends posterior and longitudinally into the calcaneal tuberosity, or a joint depressive–type fracture pattern, where the fracture exits posterior and superior to the posterior facet.[3] These fractures may also divide the anterior facet, violate the calcaneocuboid joint, and contribute to the overall comminution.

Sequelae of Calcaneal Malunions

As discussed previously, calcaneal malunions are devastating injuries resulting in significant patient morbidity. The sequelae of these injuries may include degenerative joint changes, impingement symptoms, gait alterations, and chronic pain (**Table 1**).[4–11]

CONSERVATIVE TREATMENT

The goals of nonsurgical management of calcaneal malunions are focused on optimizing patient function while minimizing discomfort. Activity modifications, such as the avoidance of ambulating on uneven grounds and limiting prolonged periods of walking, can help decrease the exacerbation of symptoms. The judicious use of anti-inflammatories or temporary immobilization may also help in disrupting the inflammatory cycle. If the pain is due to abnormal biomechanics, external support in the form of orthoses, shoe gear changes (eg, wider shoes or lace-up boots), shoe gear modifications (rocker-bottom sole), and bracing can aid in improving hindfoot alignment. Physical therapy consultations, with emphasis on gait training and the use of gait aides, can effectively limit the stresses through the symptomatic limb.

Table 1 Complications from intra-articular calcaneal malunions	
Complication	**Pathomechanics**
Ankle impingement	Loss in calcaneal height
Calcaneal varus/valgus	Translation of tuberosity fracture fragment during injury
Digital contractures	Missed compartment syndrome
Heel pain	Fat pad injury
Peroneal tendinosis/stenosis	Increased calcaneal width
Peroneal tendon subluxation/dislocation	Severe lateral calcaneal wall displacement
Posttraumatic arthrosis	Cartilage damage from initial injury, subtalar joint incongruity
Secondary arthrosis (ankle joint, midtarsal joint)	Altered hindfoot biomechanics
Subfibular impingement	Increased calcaneal width
Tibial/sural neuritis	Soft tissue scarring, traction injury, calcaneal exostosis

Data from Refs.[4–11]

Differentiating between intra-articular and neural sources of pain is best accomplished using a diagnostic injection. Typical treatments for neuritic pain include the use of pharmacologic agents as well as topical liniments. For patients with recalcitrant pain, a consultation to physical medicine and rehabilitation should also be considered. Overall, given the myriad clinical presentations, it is crucial to determine the etiology of a patient's complaint to provide the correct treatment plan.

SURGICAL TREATMENT

The decision to consider surgical management of calcaneal mal-unions follows the persistence of patient symptoms despite previous attempts at conservative cares. As surgical deformity correction is a massive undertaking with high risk for complications, patient selection is critical. Surgery should be reserved for active, motivated, and compliant patients to provide a more predictable outcome. Other considerations, such as patient age, medical comorbidities, profession, smoking status, home accessibility, and the existence of a support system, are also essential preoperative concerns. It is the responsibility of the surgeon to provide an honest discussion with the patient regarding the risks of surgery, including wound complications, infection, undercorrection or overcorrection of the deformity, need for further surgery, and the potential for limb amputation. Equally important is the emphasis of postoperative protocol and rehabilitation. Patients are to understand the prolonged period of non–weight bearing after surgery as well as the need for physical therapy to regain strength and meaningful function to the limb.

This article reviews the various procedures described in the literature for surgical treatment of calcaneal malunions. Although each selection of procedures must be patient-specific, the shared goals of surgery are to minimize pain, create a plantigrade foot, and optimize limb function.

Calcanectomy

Subtotal or complete calcanectomies are considered radical hindfoot procedures and are detailed throughout the literature. In the setting of trauma, such procedures are generally reserved for either open calcaneal fractures with extensive, complex wounding or postoperative infections, resulting in calcaneal osteomyelitis.[12] In an effort to avoid a more proximal amputation, a calcanectomy also may be considered in cases of debilitating and unsalvageable calcaneal malunion deformities. Although satisfactory outcomes after an isolated calcanectomy have been reported, the majority of the available literature suggests that patients are often left with an unstable, nonfunctional foot.[13,14] Midtarsal instability may occur after a total calcanectomy and likely require subsequent stabilization procedures with lifelong bracing.[14] In addition, the residual limb is often cosmetically displeasing and is at high risk of skin breakdown.[15] For these reasons, reconstructive procedures focusing on hindfoot preservation are typically performed after the initial calcanectomy procedure.

Calcaneal Allograft Transplantation

The use of calcaneal structural allografts has been well documented throughout the oncological literature. These reported cases generally focus on primary calcaneal tumor excision with the use of a calcaneal allograft for hindfoot reconstructive purposes. Allograft replacement has become an increasingly attractive means of restoring the weight-bearing function of the heel and allowing reattachment of the Achilles tendon apparatus. Although a technically demanding procedure, reports in the literature show promising results.

- In 1953, Ottolenghi and Petracchi[16] published one of the first studies to explore the possibility of a total calcaneal allograft transplant. A patient with chondromyxosarcoma of the calcaneus underwent a total calcanectomy and implantation of a calcaneal allograft.[16] Although the graft ultimately collapsed from reabsorption and avascular necrosis, the investigators concluded this procedure was an important advancement in hindfoot reconstructive surgery.[16]
- In a case series by Muscolo and colleagues,[17] the investigators provided 32-year follow-up and postsurgical outcomes on the original patient described by Ottolenghi and Petracchi.[16] The patient was able to ambulate pain-free without the use of a gait aid and demonstrated radiographic findings similar to those previously reported by Ottolenghi and Petracchi.[16] The second patient described by Muscolo and colleagues[17] underwent a total calcanectomy for the treatment of a giant cell tumor of the calcaneus. Replacement with a total calcaneal allograft was performed with the addition of subtalar and calcaneocuboid joint arthrodesis procedures.[17] At the 9-year follow-up, the patient was noted to have minimal pain with ambulation, and radiographs demonstrated a well-aligned heel with osseous union across the subtalar and calcaneocuboid joints.[17]
- Ayerza and colleagues[18] reported 44 allograft reconstructions, 6 of which were total calcaneal allografts. When excluding oncological complications, the overall calcaneal allograft survival rate at 5 years and 10 years postoperative was 83%.[18] Of the 6 cases, 2 revision surgeries were required (1 due to infection and the other due to graft fracture).[18] The average follow-up was 53-months, at which time all 6 calcaneal allograft patients were reportedly asymptomatic and able to bear weight.[18]
- Degeorge and colleagues[19] presented a case of a patient who underwent a total calcanectomy for management of a calcaneal chondrosarcoma. Delayed allograft reconstruction was performed using a bulk calcaneal allograft followed by subtalar and calcaneocuboid joint arthrodesis procedures.[19] At the 12-month follow-up, there was no evidence of graft necrosis or displacement (although a

subtalar joint nonunion was noted), and the patient was reportedly asymptomatic with a normal gait.[19]

Complications arising from the use of calcaneal allografts include nonunion, fracture, infection, and disease transmission. Of these complications, nonunion at the allograft-host junction is the most common, ranging from 17% to 35%.[20,21] Despite the most prevalent complication, nonunion is often less problematic than a graft fracture or infection. Delloye and colleagues[21] reviewed 128 patients who received a massive bone allograft and found 16.4% of patients developed a graft fracture and 5.4% developed a graft infection. Allograft fractures often require surgical replacement due the compromised structural integrity and risk for future collapse.[21] Deep infection is the most catastrophic complication because it necessitates explantation of the allograft and prolonged antibiotic therapy. Lastly, as with any type of allograft, there is a potential for disease transmission although this risk is minimal.

Vascularized Autograft

The use of vascularized autografts for the purpose of calcaneal restoration has been described with various types of graft compositions. Vascularized autografts are generally indicated in cases with osseous defects measuring greater than 6 cm[22] These are ideal because they provide the 3 essential elements of bone healing (osteoinduction, osteogenesis, and osteoconduction) in addition to their own vascular supply.[23] Vascularized autografts generally do not undergo resorption; they maintain their mechanical strength and readily incorporate into the donor site.[23] The vascularized autograft selection depends on the size of the osseous defect, need for soft tissue coverage, vascular status of the recipient site, and donor site morbidity.[24] Although the available literature describes multiple grafting techniques for hindfoot reconstruction after open traumatic calcaneal injuries or for the management of calcaneal tumors, vascularized autograft may also be a viable option for the treatment of unsalvageable calcaneal malunions.

Ribs

The ribs are a common donor site for vascularized free grafts; however, there are only a few cases reporting its use in hindfoot surgery. In a study by Brenner and colleagues,[24] the investigators reported a patient who sustained an open calcaneal fracture and underwent hindfoot reconstruction with vascularized double-barrel ribs and a free serratus anterior muscle flap transfer. After a subtotal calcanectomy was performed, the ribs were used to bridge the osseous defect while the serratus anterior muscle was used to fill the residual void.[24] At 5 months postoperative, the investigators noted signs of radiographic consolidation and reported good overall anatomic and functional results.[24] In a study by Yazar and colleagues,[23] the investigators reported the management of 62 patients with traumatic lower extremity injuries, 4 of which involved the calcaneus. Three of the calcaneal injuries were treated with an iliac osteocutaneous flap, whereas the remaining patient was treated with a vascularized rib and combined serratus anterior and latissimus dorsi muscle flap transfer.[23] Unfortunately, the patient who received the vascularized rib graft developed an infection that resulted in a below-knee amputation.[23]

Iliac bone crest

For the treatment of severe calcaneal injuries, the use of a vascularized iliac crest autograft is considered an ideal choice.[25] In a case series published by Peek and Giessler,[26] 1 of the presented patients was initially treated with open reduction and internal fixation of an open calcaneal fracture. The postoperative course was complicated by posterior hindfoot skin necrosis and the patient was treated with a subtotal calcanectomy.[26] A vascularized osteocutaneous iliac crest flap was used to cover the soft tissue defect and restore hindfoot function.[26] Although the recovery was complicated by flap necrosis, radiographic osseous union was achieved at 16 weeks postoperative, and the patient was able to ambulate at 8 months postoperative.[26] Similar procedures involving the use of a vascularized iliac crest graft were reported by Stevenson and colleagues,[27] Wei and colleagues,[28] and Shenaq and Dinh.[29] These investigators advocated for the use of this vascularized autograft to reconstruct the heel in the setting of traumatic calcaneal injuries.

Fibula

In opposition to rib and iliac crest free flaps, the pedicled fibular osteomyocutaneous flap provides simultaneous osseous and soft tissue reconstruction without the need for vascular anastomosis.[30] In 1995, Cai and colleagues[31] published a case series of 2 patients who sustained crush injuries to the foot. The investigators detailed the use of a vascularized, double-barreled osteomyocutaneous fibular graft pedicled on the distal peroneal vessels to recreate the heel.[31] At 6 months' follow-up, both patients had radiographic evidence of osseous union at the graft-host interface.[31] In 2010, Li and colleagues[30] retrospectively reviewed postoperative outcomes of 5 patients surgically treated for a primary calcaneal tumor. These patients underwent a total calcanectomy and a pedicled osteocutaneous fibular flap, similar to the technique described by Cai and colleagues.[31] At an average follow-up of 50.4 months, all fibular flaps survived and each patient achieved osseous union.[30] In 2012, Li and colleagues[32] published another case series of 4 patients treated for primary calcaneal tumors. These patients underwent hindfoot reconstructions with the use of a calcaneal allograft in addition to a vascularized fibular osteocutaneous flap. The average time to osseous union was 9.5 months, and revision surgery was necessary in 2 patients due to flap necrosis and infection. At final follow-up, all patients achieved successful osseous union and reported satisfactory functional outcomes. The investigators concluded that this technique exploits the mechanical stability of a calcaneal allograft while also providing an intrinsic blood supply with living cells through the vascularized fibular graft.[32]

Studies involving the use of vascularized autografts are limited to case reports and case series, thus making it difficult to compare outcomes between the various techniques and grafts. Regardless of graft composition, plastic surgery literature is replete with complications, including infection, flap necrosis, graft stress fractures, and donor site morbidity.[23] Although not specifically described for the treatment of severe calcaneal malunions, the use of vascularized autografts remain a theoretic option in cases with considerable hindfoot deformity but requires highly specialized skills not commonly performed by foot and ankle surgeons.

Calcaneal Prosthesis

The use of calcaneal prosthetic implants has been described for limb salvage procedures after surgical resection of calcaneal osseous tumors. The use of a custom calcaneal prosthesis was first documented in 1998 by Chou and Malawer.[33] The investigators performed a total calcanectomy through a posterior approach and secured the metallic calcaneal implant to the talus with screw fixation. At the 12-year follow-up, there was no reported hardware failure. The patient was able to ambulate up to 10 blocks but suffered from mild plantar heel pain.[33] In a more recent case study published by Imanishi and Choong,[34] a total calcanectomy was performed and a patient-matched 3-D calcaneal prosthesis was implanted. Using the contralateral calcaneus as a template, a custom titanium 3-D calcaneus was reconstructed with use of a specialized CT and 3-D printer. The investigators commented on several advantages of the technology, including the following: selective polishing of the prosthesis allowed for articular surface correspondence; ability for reattachment of the soft tissue structures (Achilles tendon, plantar fascia, and periarticular ligaments); meshed structure for soft tissue ingrowth capabilities; lightweight and strong design; and the short interval of time between prosthetic design to implantation. At the 5-month follow-up, the patient reportedly had satisfactory clinical results without any major complications or pain.[34]

With limited literature documenting the use of calcaneal prostheses, definitive conclusions cannot be established. Additional studies are required to assess long-term outcomes and implant survival. As technology continues to advance and custom-made implants become increasingly available to surgeons and the financial cost less prohibitive, the use of a calcaneal prosthesis may prove to be a viable treatment option in patients with unsalvageable calcaneal malunion deformities.

SUMMARY

Calcaneal malunions are a debilitating deformity that present a unique challenge to foot and ankle surgeons. Conservative management is primarily aimed at controlling symptoms and does not correct the underlying deformity. Surgical intervention is often necessary, although it is a massive undertaking and should be reserved for a select group of patients. It is of paramount importance to discuss the potential risks of surgery and manage patient expectations. The goals of calcaneal malunion surgery should be to minimize pain, create a plantigrade foot, and improve the overall function of the limb.

The majority of literature pertaining to calcaneal mal-unions is in the form of retrospective case series. Each individual deformity is unique from others, making comparison studies difficult to design. Furthermore, with regard to treating unsalvageable calcaneal malunions, limited literature exists. Treatment options, such as calcanectomy, calcaneal allograft transplantation, vascularized autograft reconstruction, and use of a calcaneal prosthesis, are extrapolated from the infectious disease, plastic surgery, and oncological literature. As technology continues to advance, there will be a need for further research regarding the use and longevity of these treatments. The available literature on the aforementioned reconstructive procedures, however, shows promise in the treatment of severe calcaneal malunion deformities.

REFERENCES

1. Reddy V, Fukuda T, Ptaszek AJ. Calcaneus malunion and nonunion. Foot Ankle Clin N Am 2007;12:125–35.
2. Atkins RM. The treatment of calcaneal malunion. Foot Ankle Clin N Am 2014;19: 521–40.
3. Maskill JD, Bohay DR, Anderson JG. Calcaneus fractures: a review article. Foot Ankle Clin N Am 2005;10:463–89.
4. Ball ST, Jadin K, Allen RT, et al. Chondrocyte viability after intra-articular calcaneal fractures in humans. Foot Ankle Int 2007;28:665–8.
5. Borrelli J Jr, Torzilli PA, Grigiene R, et al. Effect of impact load on articular cartilage: development of an intra-articular fracture model. J Orthop Trauma 1997; 11:319–26.
6. Stapleton JJ, Belczyk R, Zgonis T. Surgical treatment of calcaneal fracture malunions and posttraumatic deformities. Clin Podiatr Med Surg 2009;26:79–90.

7. Mulcahy DM, McCormack DM, Stephens MM. Intra-articular calcaneal fractures: effect of open reduction and internal fixation on the contact characteristics of the subtalar joint. Foot Ankle Int 1998;19:842–8.

8. Banerjee R, Saltzman C, Anderson RB, et al. Management of calcaneal malunion. J Am Acad Orthop Surg 2011;19:27–36.

9. Howard JL, Buckley R, McCormack R, et al. Complications following management of displaced intra-articular calcaneal fractures: a prospective randomized trial comparing open reduction internal fixation with nonoperative management. J Orthop Trauma 2003;17:241–9.

10. Clare MP, Crawford WS. Managing complications of calcaneus fractures. Foot Ankle Clin N Am 2017;22:105–16.

11. Saltzman CL, El-Khoury GY. The hindfoot alignment view. Foot Ankle Int 1995;16: 572–6.

12. Oznur A, Komurcu M, Marangoz S, et al. A new perspective on management of open calcaneus fractures. Int Orthop 2008;32:785–90.

13. Dhillon M, Singh B, Gil S, et al. Management of giant cell tumor of the tarsal bones: a report of nine cases and a review of the literature. Foot Ankle 1993; 14:265–72.

14. Baumhauer JF, Fraga CJ, Gould JS, et al. Total calcanectomy for the treatment of chronic calcaneal osteomyelitis. Foot Ankle Int 1998;19:849–55.

15. Smith DG, Stuck RM, Ketner L, et al. Partial calcanectomy for the treatment of large ulceration of the heel and calcaneal osteomyelitis. An amputation of the back of the foot. J Bone Joint Surg Am 1992;74:571–6.

16. Ottolenghi CE, Petracchi LJ. Chondromyxosarcoma of the calcaneus: report of a case of total replacement of involved bone with a homogenous refrigerated calcaneus. J Bone Joint Surg Am 1953;35:211–4.

17. Muscolo DL, Ayerza MA, Aponte-Tinao LA. Long-term results of allograft replacement after total calcanectomy: a report of two cases. J Bone Joint Surg Am 2000; 82:109–12.

18. Ayerza MA, Piuzzi NS, Aponte-Tinao LA, et al. Structural allograft reconstruction of the foot and ankle after tumor resections. Musculoskelet Surg 2016;100: 149–56.

19. Degeorge B, Dagneaux L, Forget D, et al. Delayed reconstruction by total calcaneal allograft following calcanectomy: is it an option? Case Rep Orthop 2016; 2016:4012180.

20. Donati D, Di Bella C, Col Angeli M, et al. The use of massive bone allografts in bone tumor surgery of the limb. Curr Orthop 2005;19:393–9.

21. Delloye C, Van Cauter M, Dufrane D, et al. Local complications of massive bone allografts: an appraisal of their prevalence in 128 patients. Acta Orthop Belg 2014;80:196–204.

22. Taylor GI, Miller GD, Ham FJ. The free vascularized bone graft a clinical extension of microvascular techniques. Plast Reconstr Surg 1975;55:533–44.

23. Yazar S, Lin CH, Wei FC. One-stage reconstruction of composite bone and soft-tissue defects in traumatic lower extremities. Plast Reconstr Surg 2004;114: 1457–66.

24. Brenner P, Zwipp H, Rammelt S. Vascularized double barrel ribs combined with free serratus anterior muscle transfer for homologous restoration of the hindfoot after calcanectomy. J Trauma 2000;49:331–5.

25. Scoccianti G, Campanacci DA, Innocenti M, et al. Total calcanectomy and reconstruction with vascularized iliac bone graft for osteoblastoma: a report of two cases. Foot Ankle Int 2009;30:716–20.

26. Peek A, Giessler GA. Functional total and subtotal heel reconstruction with free composite osteofasciocutaneous groin flap of the deep circumflex iliac vessels. Ann Plast Surg 2006;56:628–34.
27. Stevenson TR, Greene TL, Kling TF Jr. Heel reconstruction with the deep circumflex iliac artery osteocutaneous flap. Plast Reconstr Surg 1987;79:982–6.
28. Wei FC, Chen HC, Chuang CC, et al. Reconstruction of achilles tendon and calcaneus defects with skin-aponeurosis-bone composite free tissue from the groin region. Plast Reconstr Surg 1988;81:579–89.
29. Shenaq SM, Dinh TA. Heel reconstruction with an iliac osteocutaneous free flap in a child. Microsurgery 1989;10:93–8.
30. Li J, Guo Z, Pei GX, et al. Limb salvage surgery for calcaneal malignancy. J Surg Oncol 2010;102:48–53.
31. Cai J, Cao X, Liang J, et al. Heel reconstruction. Plast Reconstr Surg 1997;99: 448–53.
32. Li J, Wang Z, Guo Z, et al. Composite biological reconstruction following total calcanectomy of primary calcaneal tumors. J Surg Oncol 2012;105:673–8.
33. Chou LB, Malawer MM. Osteosarcoma of the calcaneus treated with prosthetic replacement with twelve years of followup: a case report. Foot Ankle Int 2007; 28:841–4.
34. Imanishi J, Choong PF. Three-dimensional printed calcaneal prosthesis following total calcanectomy. Int J Surg Case Rep 2015;10:83–7.

Moving?

Make sure your subscription moves with you!

To notify us of your new address, find your **Clinics Account Number** (located on your mailing label above your name), and contact customer service at:

Email: journalscustomerservice-usa@elsevier.com

800-654-2452 (subscribers in the U.S. & Canada)
314-447-8871 (subscribers outside of the U.S. & Canada)

Fax number: 314-447-8029

Elsevier Health Sciences Division
Subscription Customer Service
3251 Riverport Lane
Maryland Heights, MO 63043

*To ensure uninterrupted delivery of your subscription, please notify us at least 4 weeks in advance of move.